Losing the last 5 kilos

Michelle Bridges has worked in the fitness industry for eighteen years as a professional trainer and group fitness instructor. Her role as a trainer on Channel Ten's hit reality weight-loss show *The Biggest Loser* has made her Australia's most recognised personal trainer. Michelle has travelled the world presenting at global fitness conventions and competing in physique and fitness competitions, and is sought after as a motivational speaker. ***Losing the Last 5 Kilos*** is her third book. Her first two, ***Crunch Time*** and ***Crunch Time Cookbook***, were bestsellers.

michellebridges.com.au

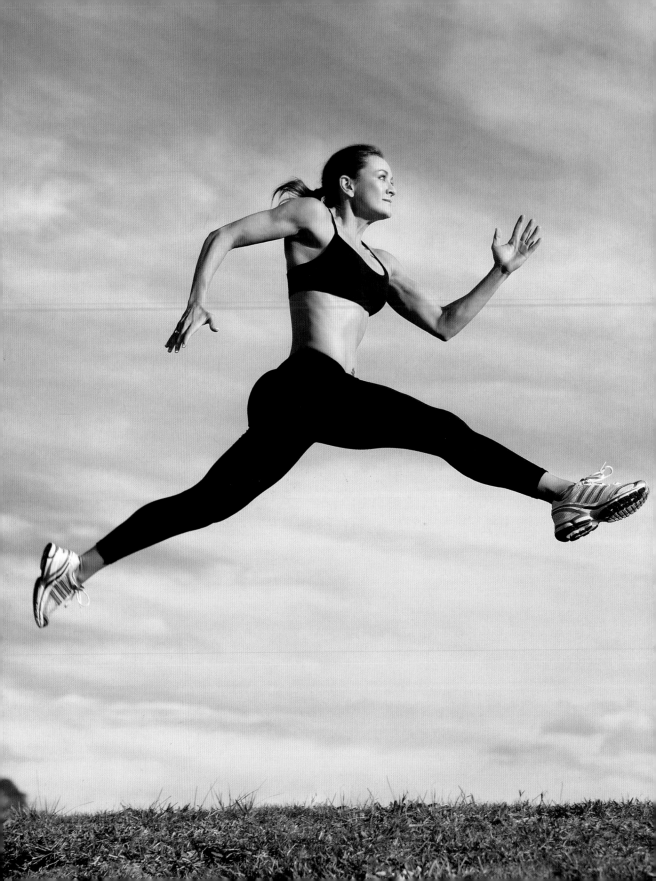

Losing
the last
5 kilos

your *kick-arse* guide to
looking & feeling *fantastic*

michelle bridges

VIKING
an imprint of
PENGUIN BOOKS

VIKING

Published by the Penguin Group
Penguin Group (Australia)
250 Camberwell Road, Camberwell, Victoria 3124, Australia
(a division of Pearson Australia Group Pty Ltd)
Penguin Group (USA) Inc.
375 Hudson Street, New York, New York 10014, USA
Penguin Group (Canada)
90 Eglinton Avenue East, Suite 700, Toronto, Canada ON M4P 2Y3
(a division of Pearson Penguin Canada Inc.)
Penguin Books Ltd
80 Strand, London WC2R 0RL, England
Penguin Ireland
25 St Stephen's Green, Dublin 2, Ireland
(a division of Penguin Books Ltd)
Penguin Books India Pvt Ltd
11 Community Centre, Panchsheel Park, New Delhi – 110 017, India
Penguin Group (NZ)
67 Apollo Drive, Rosedale, North Shore 0632, New Zealand
(a division of Pearson New Zealand Ltd)
Penguin Books (South Africa) (Pty) Ltd
24 Sturdee Avenue, Rosebank, Johannesburg 2196, South Africa

Penguin Books Ltd, Registered Offices: 80 Strand, London WC2R 0RL, England

First published by Penguin Group (Australia), 2011

10 9 8 7 6 5 4 3

Cover and text design by Adam Laszczuk © Penguin Group (Australia)
Exercise photography by Nick Wilson
Photography on pages 12, 25, 26, 58 by Rob Palmer
Food photography by Lisa Cohen
Styling by Deb Kaloper
Food preparation by Tony Chiodo
Food consultant Lucy Nunes
Typeset in Gotham Narrow by Post Pre-Press Group, Brisbane, Queensland
Colour reproduction by Splitting Image, Clayton, Victoria
Printed in China by 1010 Printing International Ltd

National Library of Australia
Cataloguing-in-Publication data:

Bridges, Michelle.
Losing the last 5 kilos / Michelle Bridges
9780670074815 (pbk.)
Weight loss
Reducing exercises
Reducing diets

613.712

penguin.com.au

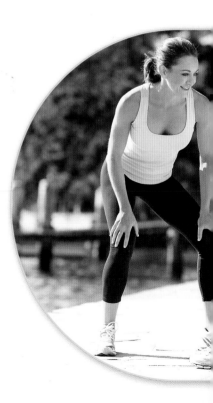

The publishers would like to thank Mandalay Designs (mandalaydesigns.com.au),
Market Import (marketimport.com) and Southwood Trading (southwoodhome.com.au).

Contents

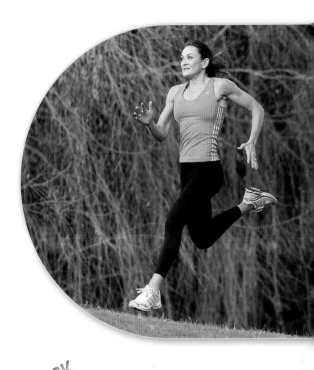

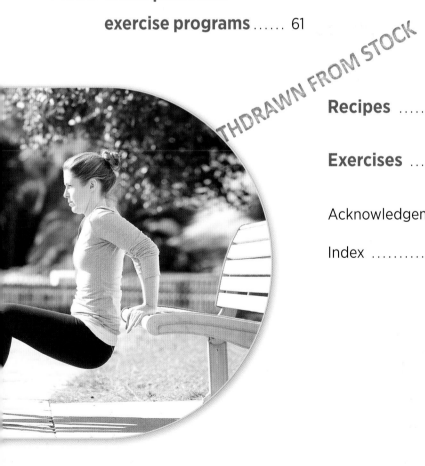

CHANCES ARE YOU'VE PICKED UP THIS BOOK because you're sick to death of lugging around those extra kilos and you want to look and feel better. Maybe you've just had a baby, or the middle-age spread has snuck up on you, or you've lost a lot of weight already but can't get the last five off. Or maybe you are desperate to get into your skinny jeans (or just any jeans!). Whatever the reason, my first question to you is 'Where is this on your list of priorities?' Because I'm here to tell ya, honey, if it ain't high enough on that list, then it ain't gonna happen. Dropping those last kilos must be a *high* priority.

Why? Because it takes commitment, focus and discipline. Do you think that Jennifer Hawkins just turns up looking the way she does? Or that all those Hollywood actors are just born lucky? Are you kidding? Tenacity and self-discipline *drive* these boys and girls.

So the bottom line is, if you want a killer bottom line, then you will have to work for it.

The good news is that I have trained enough people in my time to know exactly what you need to do to achieve this. In Part 1, I talk about why those last 5 kilos are so stubborn, and why you have been struggling to get them off. Getting your head around the science of what happens to your body and mind is the first step to taking back control. Once you understand *why* the last 5 kilos are so hard to lose, you'll understand why your old strategies (e.g. skipping meals, playing mind games) never worked, and what you need to do to ensure success.

In Part 2, I give you all the ammo you'll need to drop those last stubborn kilos in just 30 days. This not only includes a day-by-day meal and exercise plan, but also detailed descriptions of my favourite low-calorie recipes and killer exercises.

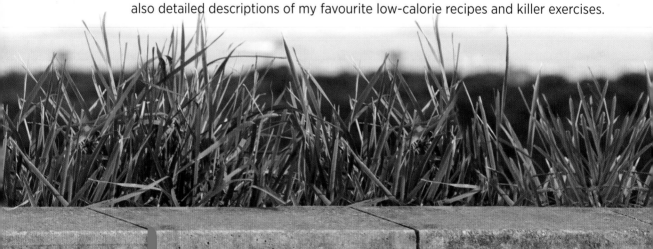

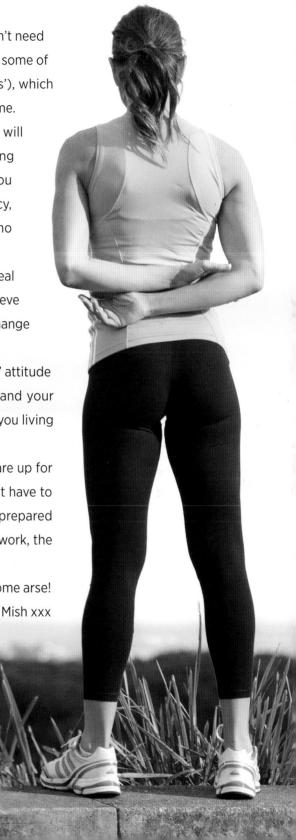

I even give you a weekly shopping list so that you don't need to think, you just have to do. I'm also letting you in on some of my special training secrets (such as 'accelerator days'), which will have you slimming down and shaping up in no time.

Knowledge is power, and that's what this book will give you in spades. For the next month you are going to take 100 per cent, total responsibility for what you do or don't put in your mouth, and for the consistency, intensity and content of your training. No blame, no victim mentality. Just do it.

So here's my promise to you: if you follow my meal plan and exercise program to the letter, you will achieve what you desire. If you don't follow it, nothing will change for you. It's really that simple.

Preparation, consistency and a 'take no prisoners' attitude are mandatory, so bring your notepad, your diary and your inner shit-kicker with you and together we will have you living out your wildest imaginings!

If you have read this far, then I am thinking you are up for it. You don't have to be a seasoned athlete; you don't have to be the most genetically gifted. You just have to be prepared to do the work. As the saying goes, 'The harder you work, the luckier you get.'

Let's kick some arse!

Mish xxx

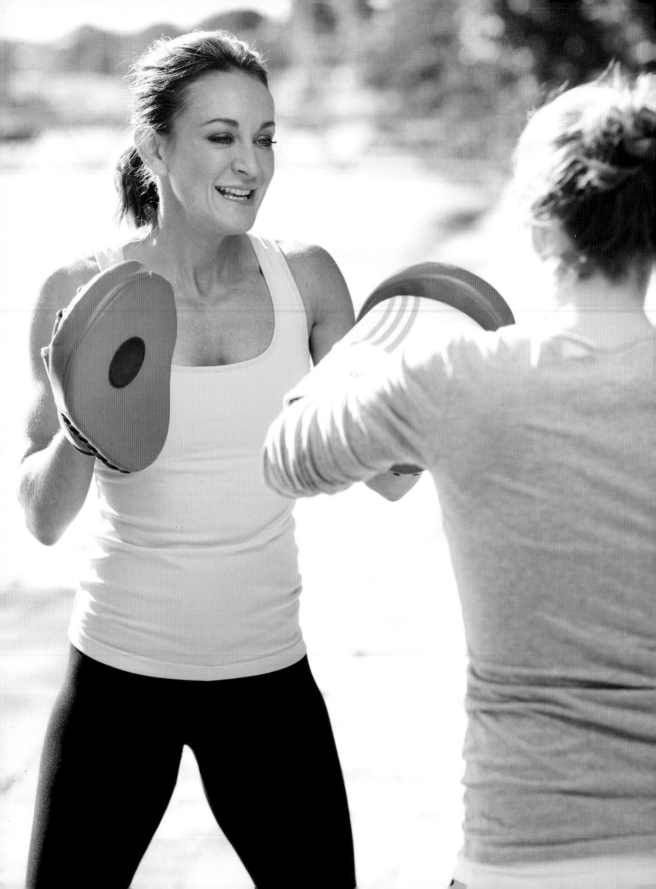

the last 5 kilos

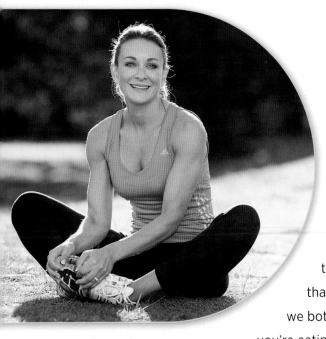

Why it's so hard to lose 5 kilos

OKAY. WE BOTH KNOW WHY you're reading this book – you want to lose the extra kilos that are between you and your ideal weight. And we both know **the main reason** those kilos are there: you're eating more calories than you burn. Eat more than you burn, you put on weight. Burn more than you eat, you lose it.

I've always been blown away by how much exercise you have to do to work off calories: for example, a regular cappuccino (100 calories) and a berry muffin (500 calories) will take a 60-minute jog to burn off; a glass of wine (120 calories) will take the equivalent of a 2 km power walk. Just having a daily muffin and coffee will give you an extra 3000 calories a week. When you consider that around 7000 calories equates to a gross weight gain of almost a kilogram, and add those extra calories to no exercise, it's not hard to see why you're going up a clothing size every year.

As you know, I'm a massive fan of exercise – it does amazing things for your mind, body and spirit – but I have to be completely honest here: **losing weight will always come down to what you put in your mouth; end of story**. If I had two clients, one of whom ate whatever she liked but I trained her like a demon, and another who did no exercise but tidied up her diet so she had a weekly calorie deficit, **the non-exerciser would lose the most weight**. Of course, the best scenario is the double-whammy: good nutrition PLUS exercise and that's what I'm giving you in the 30-day plan. You don't even need to count your calories – I do it all for you, so you can focus on getting organised and staying committed.

'But . . .' I hear you protest, 'I've been eating salad, saying no to dessert and exercising and **I still can't lose the last 5 kilos!** There's something you're not telling me!' And you're right. It's a bit more complicated if you've already lost a stack of weight, are a bit older or have had a baby. Sometimes our bodies actually **work against us** losing those last few kilos.

How our bodies work against us

Anyone who watches *The Biggest Loser* will know that the contestants' weight losses in the first few weeks are freaky – some of these guys and girls strip off 1 or even 2 kilos *a day* as their bodies respond to consistent, intense exercise and clean eating. Even some participants on my Twelve Week Body Transformation (check it out at www.12wbt.com) drop 3 or 4 kilos in the first few days, and that's without me reducing them to tears twice a day for two hours! So when it comes down to the last 5 kilos that simply don't seem to want to come off, you could be forgiven for getting just a teensy bit frustrated.

But the reason is pretty straightforward, really: **moving a 120-kilogram body takes a lot more energy than moving an 80-kilogram body**, so in the space of any given time the energy expenditure will always be more. All that extra movement needs fuel, and body fat is perfect for the job. Muscle needs plenty of energy to sustain itself, a lot more than fat – around nine times more, in fact. So working muscles hard by moving around a body weighed down with heaps of body fat means that you can smash a *lot* of calories in your workouts.

Some of the big boys in *The Biggest Loser* house would regularly burn off 1200 or more calories in the space of just one hour's training, which is huge when you consider they're only eating about 1800–1900 calories for the day (that drops to 1600 later on). By comparison, I'm happy to burn off 600 calories in a one-hour session, and I keep my calories at around 1200–1300 per day. Of course, as you become **lighter and fitter**, your muscles don't have to work quite so hard, and your calorie-burning capacity reduces.

But there is another important reason why our weight loss slows down, and it has to do with our biological survival. Think about it: if there were no mechanism for human beings to re-establish the energy in/energy out balance, we would simply keep losing weight until we shrivelled up and died.

Our bodies are cleverly constructed to stop this from happening, and here's how it works. If you simply cut your daily calorie intake over the course of a few weeks you will gradually lose weight. This is because your body still needs the same amount of energy to keep you moving, and so it sources this energy from stored fat. However, it doesn't only source it from fat stores (it needs to keep some for emergencies), so it also breaks down protein, which means that you are also gradually losing some lean muscle.

As your lean muscle gradually reduces, so does your metabolic rate, and with it your energy requirements. (This is why I am so adamant that you must retain your lean muscle by weight training and refuelling your body with sufficient lean protein.) At some point in your weight loss, your calorie deficit will become so small that **your body no longer recognises that it needs to burn stored body fat.** The balance has been restored. Your body no longer thinks that there is a calorie deficit – which is great if we're roaming the Jurassic savannah searching for food, but not much fun when we're lying on the bed with our legs in the air trying to get into a pair of jeans that have just come out of the dryer.

The combination of a reduced overall energy expenditure (because we're lighter) and a reduction in our muscle mass (because we've been nibbling away at the proteins that make it up) means that **those last 5 kilos are the hardest ones of all for us to lose**.

Get it?

'It must be my metabolism'

But what about people who have **always been half a dozen kilos overweight** and just can't seem to lose them? I've often heard these people talking about fast and slow metabolisms. You know the kind of café chat: 'Oh, my husband can eat anything and he never puts on weight, he's got such a fast metabolism', or 'I've got a really slow metabolism. I only have to look at a hamburger to put on 2 kilos.' Now let's take this apart.

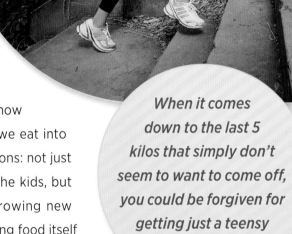

Put simply, our metabolic rate determines how quickly, or how slowly, we convert the food we eat into the fuel that allows our bodies to perform actions: not just running, mowing the lawn and playing with the kids, but basic bodily functions such as breathing, growing new cells, and perspiring. Even the action of digesting food itself requires energy.

When it comes down to the last 5 kilos that simply don't seem to want to come off, you could be forgiven for getting just a teensy bit frustrated.

So what determines our metabolic rate? There is a genetic component, of course, plus our age, and whether we live in a cold or warm climate. However, it's **the amount of lean muscle** we carry that will have the most profound effect on our metabolism – that, and the amount of fat we carry. Add some muscle, drop some fat, and our metabolic rate goes up.

It isn't that complicated. In fact, it's pretty bloody simple. **Our metabolic rates are largely determined by our lifestyles**.

Alarm bells start ringing whenever I hear that 'groundbreaking scientific discoveries' are said to have unravelled the mystery of why we're all getting fat. These discoveries usually have three characteristics in common: firstly, you don't have to actually do any exercise to lose weight; secondly, they are complex and use a lot of big words; and thirdly (and here's the clincher) you usually have to hand over your credit-card number or you'll never learn the 'secret' to avoiding a lifetime of self-loathing and fatness.

I reckon I'm a bit of a scientist. In fact, my time training people has been like one huge experiment. I've spent thousands of hours training hundreds and hundreds of people. All kinds of people: fat people, thin people, old people. And I'm here to tell you that **I have discovered the secret!** The secret that has eluded generations of scientists, intellectuals and academics . . .

Eat less, move more.

Pretty complex, eh? By eating less, I don't mean starving yourself. If you starve yourself you will lose weight, but as we've seen, your body is biologically geared to switch to survival mode when there is less food around and it lowers your metabolism by eating away at your precious muscle mass as well as your fat stores. I've also seen it many times: people starve themselves and then they binge. **It never works.**

'It must be my genes'

The excuse that you can't lose weight because you have 'bad genes' actually falls into a similar category as the excuse that you've been cursed with a slow metabolism by those lousy parents of yours. To put it bluntly, **there is no 'fat gene'**. Sorry, but there just isn't.

In the past, it was accepted that the genes we inherited from our parents would determine all of our physical characteristics. This is still partly true, but scientists now know that a significant proportion of our health and physical characteristics are determined by our lifestyle (what we do, what we eat, etc) – around two-thirds, in fact. The rest is hardwired in our genetics. This means that **how we live** will have by far the greatest influence on **how we look** and **how healthy we are**.

So if you're overweight, it's not because of your genes, it's because of the **way you have treated them**. In season five of *The Biggest Loser* we made the contestants run a marathon. Now if you've ever done any running, you'd know what a tough proposition that is. In training for the marathon, the contestants (one of whom was unable to *walk* 500 metres) went from physiological basket cases on day one to completing 42 gruelling kilometres just four months later. Their genes hadn't changed, but everything else had – their lean muscle mass, body fat level and cardiovascular fitness. **They were physiologically different**.

You may think that you're stuck with your body. You're not. Some of us believe that those last 5 kilos will never come off. They will!

> I really learnt to recognise the signs of my emotional eating and how not to indulge in these patterns. I have learnt some valuable lessons and feel I am far better able to cope and work around these issues instead of falling down in a mess.
>
> *Kate, 27, Brisbane*

'Super' sugar

The average Australian consumes 22 teaspoons of sugar a day! Most of this is hidden sugar – fructose. So the main reason for our obesity crisis is not the fats in our diet, but rather the amount of **sugar** we now consume.

Everyday table sugar (sucrose) comprises 50 per cent glucose and 50 per cent fructose. Glucose is our body's primary energy source and can be metabolised by many parts of our bodies – our brain, our kidneys, our muscles – but fructose can only be metabolised by our liver, which causes all sorts of problems.

Fructose is everywhere these days, being the preferred sweetener in so-called 'sugar-free' or 'low-cal' products (think diet soft drinks, diet yoghurts, diet cordials). We even make a 'super' sugar – high-fructose corn syrup – which is cheap, super sweet and gets added to all kinds of foods and drinks, particularly soft drinks. But our body was never designed to consume such a massive amount of fructose – particularly as it's left to our poor old liver to do all the metabolising, which, by the way, is usually overloaded by virtue of the modern world's toxic lifestyle (think alcohol, caffeine, medication etc.).

Overloading our liver with fructose does a lot of bad things to them, but most significantly it shuts down their insulin receptors, meaning that **our bodies think that we need more insulin**, when in fact we're swimming in the stuff! And what does excess insulin do? Among other things, it makes us fat.

Here's how it works. Every time we eat, the hormone insulin is released into our bloodstream from special cells in the pancreas. The insulin encourages our tissues – especially our muscles – to guzzle up the glucose surging through our bloodstream after we eat a meal, which is cool, because glucose hanging around in the blood is dangerous stuff. It interferes with proteins and in the long term can result in diabetes which can lead to kidney damage, blindness and even amputation. The insulin rushes around looking for the glucose and stores it as glycogen in our liver and muscles. But our bodies can only store enough glycogen for one active day. So once we have filled up our glycogen stores, that **sugar is stored as saturated fat**.

This fructose bombardment also increases our blood pressure and loads us up with the bad form of cholesterol. So look out for 'high fructose corn syrup' or 'sucrose' on the labels of processed or packaged foods (which you should be steering clear of anyway). While the rest of the label might say 'low fat' or 'fat-free', the fructose–insulin effect means you will still end up building your fat stores,

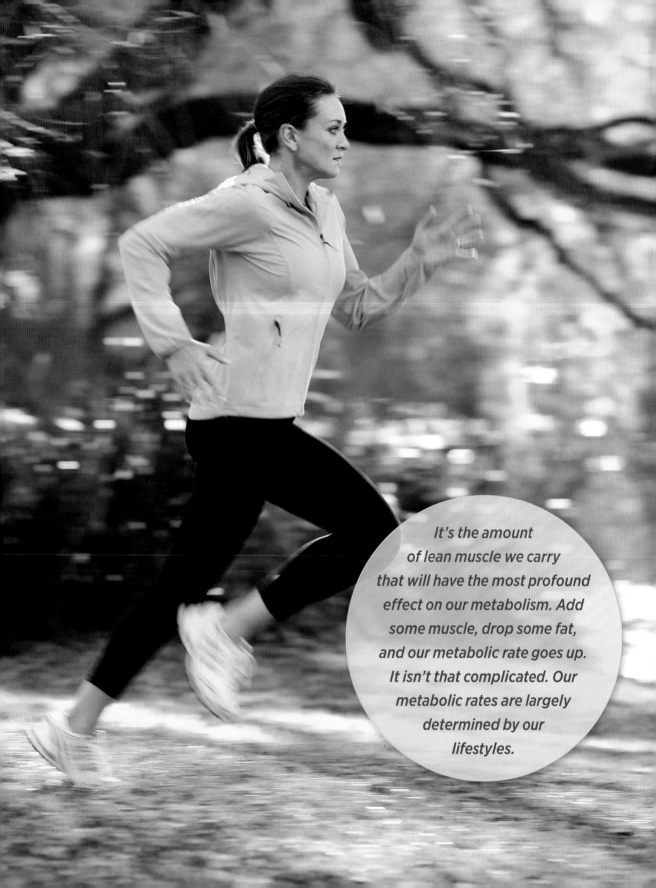

It's the amount of lean muscle we carry that will have the most profound effect on our metabolism. Add some muscle, drop some fat, and our metabolic rate goes up. It isn't that complicated. Our metabolic rates are largely determined by our lifestyles.

especially when, if you are honest with yourself, you always end up eating more when you think it's fat-free!

> There aren't enough words that I can say to express my immense gratitude to Mish for helping set me on a fit and health path for life. Since training with her, my life motto is 'Consistent hard work = results!' I'm now a healthy, fit size 12 (literally half my size) and living my life to the max, every single day!

Amiee, 27, Sydney

The joys of ageing

Have you ever noticed that most of us seem to get gradually bigger and bigger as we get older? That only a handful of us seem to stay in control of our weight over the years and that the rest of us just seem to be forever expanding?

Now before we start getting all sensitive about the word 'old', just know that even if *we* don't think we're getting old, these bodies of ours *do.* In fact, from our early twenties we quietly begin to deteriorate. We tell ourselves, 'Oh, well. I'm not as young as I used to be,' or 'I never really lost my baby weight.' But the fact is that most of the time **our lifestyles are responsible for us losing control.** As we get older we become more sedentary and less active. Plus we've often got more time to hang around cafés and eat out and we usually have a lot more disposable income. But there's also a biological reason why we get heavier. It's because from the age of around twenty-five our metabolism – the chemical process that converts food to energy – starts to slow down.

Slowed metabolism

If we think of our body as a car engine, our metabolism is literally the size of the engine. We all start life as a V8 and gradually fade to a four-cylinder as we age, reducing our fuel-burning capacity.

So you can see the problem here: our bodies and our lifestyles are conspiring against us at two levels. **Not only are we eating more calories**, but we're also reducing our ability to burn them because we have less lean muscle!

We can even find ourselves in the bizarre situation of actually getting fatter without getting heavier. Muscle weighs more than fat, so you can lose muscle and gain fat without any change to your weight. And if you don't keep using your muscles they will simply shrink until the day comes when you open your 'garage door' to find a Smart Car where your V8 Supercar used to be parked!

Falling hormone levels

As we age, we not only lose muscle tone by living a more sedentary lifestyle, but because the production of hormones that support muscle growth (such as testosterone in men) slows down. Unfortunately for all you blokes out there, testosterone levels start slipping from around the age of 30 at the rate of about 1 per cent a year, or even more if you have any testicular damage.

But before us girls start getting too smug, there's a ton of research showing that as our oestrogen levels fall, our metabolic rates fall too, and with them our calorie-burning ability. So we can be eating the **same number of calories** and even doing the same amount of exercise as we did before we reached middle age, but we still put on weight. The only thing that actually increases is our appetite (seriously! See page 14). Aaaargh! Is this not proof that God is a man?!

Falling oestrogen levels also mess with our glucose tolerance – how our bodies cope with sugar. This perfect storm of female fatness turns up significantly after menopause (usually at around 50).

One mind-blowing moment for me was when I read about another senior managing to run 400 metres, and I thought how hard this had been for me but I had done it, then I read more and realised the senior was 90 years old. I threw out my ageist attitude and I just went at the challenge as if I were 20 years old.

Kathy, 64, Melbourne

Sara Visser

Straight after my marriage I went from being fit and lean to fluctuating between 5 and 10 kilograms over my ideal weight. I kept hoping that my one session a week with my personal trainer would magically get me back to my ideal weight. When I started to dislike looking in the mirror and refusing to have my photo taken, I realised it was time to take action.

Thanks to Michelle's program, I finally found the focus and drive that had been missing over the past five years. I unlearnt old habits, set firm goals to achieve and stopped making excuses not to exercise. In twelve weeks I lost 8.4 kilograms and am honestly the fittest, healthiest and happiest I have ever been.

Increased appetite

Not satisfied with ripping off our precious hormones, nature also ups the ante by trying to make us eat more as we get older.

Research by scientists at Monash University has shown that the cells that control our appetite are gradually damaged over time, mostly when we're aged 25 to 30. Appetite-controlling cells (POMC neurons) are progressively damaged and killed off by free radicals as we get older, so while our hunger neurons are still relaying the message that we're hungry, the ones relaying the message that our hunger is satisfied become impaired, and we're in the kitchen helping ourselves to seconds.

The most significant damage takes place after we've been tucking into foods that are rich in – you guessed it! – refined or processed carbohydrates and sugars (in other words, junk or fast food), the same food group that has been almost single-handedly responsible for our obesity epidemic (along with its podgy little mate, fat).

Too much fat in our midsection can fast-track us to lifestyle diseases such as atherosclerosis and diabetes, which are not only debilitating but life-threatening – all the more reason to eat less and move more.

The effects of stress

When we are under stress, our adrenal gland pumps out adrenaline (the 'fight or flight' hormone that elevates heart rate, blood pressure and respiration) and cortisol, which is involved in glucose metabolism and blood sugar maintenance (to supply the energy we need) as well as inflammatory response and immune function.

Unlike adrenaline, which is only produced in short bursts, cortisol can be produced long term. And one of the things an elevated cortisol level does is to increase abdominal fat. From a survival point of view, this emergency fat storage is designed to keep a person alive if they have to endure harsh or physically demanding conditions for long periods. The problem is, we're leading sedentary lives (driving cars and sitting in offices) and much of the stress is in our heads. Our modern way of life means that our cortisol level gets pumped up so many times during our busy day that it doesn't get much chance to return to normal, and most of us aren't burning any of the extra fat that's being stored in the process. Too much fat in our midsection can fast-track us to lifestyle diseases such as atherosclerosis and diabetes, which are not only debilitating but life-threatening – all the more reason to eat less and move more. Oh, and on the topic of stress, there's a huge amount of research to prove that exercise substantially reduces anxiety and depression. **Hello? Can anyone hear me out there?!**

Baby weight

So far we've looked at how metabolism, age, diet and stress work together to make it hard to shift the last 5 kilos. Post-pregnancy weight can also be hard to shift, and is the reason many women give for being overweight. And of course it takes some time to get back to your ideal weight after having a baby. However, I am sick of hearing about Hollywood stars who look 'radiant' after losing their baby weight in just one week. Let me tell you how she got the weight off. She had a nanny for the baby and a personal trainer **to flog her** in the gym for three hours twice a day, ate one carrot a day for two weeks, and then posed for some careful shots that went straight to the retouching lab.

You can get back to your pre-pregnancy weight quite quickly, but don't do it in a way that is going to stress you out. You've just had a baby, remember! Although I'm a rapid weight loss fan, the introduction of a new human being to the world – **your human being** – would have to be one instance where I wouldn't recommend ripping yourself back into shape the morning after. There is even some evidence that environmental toxins stored in body fat may be released into breast milk if weight is shed too quickly after childbirth.

Start off on the right foot

The best way to lose baby weight is to **start before you conceive**. Set yourself up for success by being your optimum weight from day one, and so shoot for a body mass index (BMI) of between 20 and 25 (check out www.michellebridges.com to calculate your BMI if you're not sure) and a body fat level of around 25 per cent.

Yep. That's right: *25* per cent. I know for some of you that might seem a lot, but when it comes to body fat percentage, there's a fair bit of nonsense flying around too. Most women actually stop menstruating if their body fat levels fall to 17 or 18 per cent because their bodies aren't convinced that there's enough stored energy to see them through a pregnancy, let alone the breastfeeding. It's our body's way of safeguarding us and our babies.

Recent studies have shown that if you begin your pregnancy overweight, you are not only more likely to **put on excess weight during pregnancy**, but you're also going to find it harder to lose weight afterwards, so getting off on the right foot is doubly important.

When I was pregnant I had gestational diabetes and needed to inject myself with insulin three times a day. Women with gestational diabetes are at increased risk of developing Type 2 diabetes and being severely obese contributes to the risk. By reducing my weight, training and eating well, I am doing everything I can to reduce the risk.

Amanda, 41, Sydney

The case for good nutrition

Think about it: could there be a more critical period in your nutritional life than when you're carrying a baby? More and more research suggests that the type of food you eat during pregnancy plays an important role in your unborn child's life. Studies have linked fatty, sugary diets in overweight mothers to the development of obesity, diabetes and even behavioural disorders in their offspring. One pregnant woman I met told me she felt fine about indulging her daily family-block-of-chocolate fetish because pregnancy was the one time she could 'let herself go'. When I put it to her that the food she was eating was playing a direct role in the growth and development of her unborn child, she soon changed her mind. A little bit of chocolate here or there is fine, but not half a kilo of the stuff!

During pregnancy, **you are helping to establish the blueprint** of your child's physiological development. So the next time you're thinking about 'eating for two', steer your pregnant self away from the greasy fries and towards the wholegrain salad sandwich. If you need to, use the power of positive language. Replace 'eating for two' with '**make what you eat count for twice as much**' and you'll be okay.

Of course, your influence goes way beyond pregnancy and babyhood. Children don't begin to develop fat cells until the age of six, but overweight children start developing them from the age of two, and continue to do so, along with normal weight children, until the end of puberty. So while the *number* of fat cells remains constant in adulthood (they enlarge when we put weight on and shrink when we lose it), an overweight child can be burdened with up to 50 per cent more fat cells than other children, and once you've got 'em, you've got 'em for life.

The message here is loud and clear. Feed your growing children healthy food (no salty, sugary junk) or you will be setting them up for a lifetime of weight and health issues and all the heartache, frustration and emotional roller-coaster baggage that comes with them.

The next step to returning to your pre-pregnancy weight is to make sure that you don't pile on the weight **during** your pregnancy. Most women put on a couple of kilos in the first trimester, and the weight gain from that point forward is usually evenly spread at around half a kilo a week, with perhaps a little more towards the end.

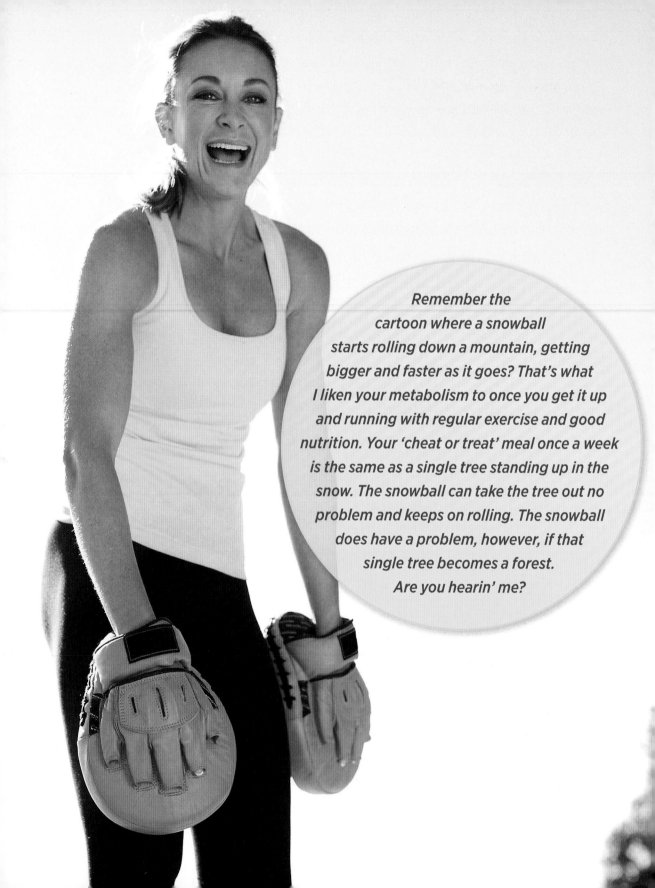

Remember the cartoon where a snowball starts rolling down a mountain, getting bigger and faster as it goes? That's what I liken your metabolism to once you get it up and running with regular exercise and good nutrition. Your 'cheat or treat' meal once a week is the same as a single tree standing up in the snow. The snowball can take the tree out no problem and keeps on rolling. The snowball does have a problem, however, if that single tree becomes a forest.
Are you hearin' me?

Importantly, your weight gain should be slower if you are overweight than if you are underweight. Check out the table below as a guide, and you'll see what I mean.

BMI	Recommended Weight Gain
30+	5–9 kgs (11–20 lbs)
25–29.9	7–11 kgs (15–25 lbs)
18.6–24.9	11–16 kgs (25–35 lbs)
18.5 and lower	13–18 kgs (28–40 lbs)

It's time to flex your willpower muscle! Your willpower is exactly like a muscle, so the more you use it, the stronger it becomes. So get it working!

This means that for a woman with a BMI of 30 or more (technically obese), total weight gain through-out the pregnancy should pretty much be accounted for by the weight of the baby, the amniotic fluid he or she is bobbing around in, and any additional weight due to lactation.

By contrast, an underweight woman **needs to be gaining body fat** during the pregnancy – breastfeeding can chew up approximately 300–600 calories a day – so getting to a good pre-conception weight is equally important if you're underweight.

Breastfeeding uses up fat that has been stored through pregnancy, so there is some biochemical sense to the idea of 'breastfeeding the baby weight away'. In fact, some studies have shown that breastfeeding mothers tend to lose more weight when their babies are three to six months old than formula-feeding mothers who are actually consuming fewer calories, so it's got to be your first choice. However, weight loss while breastfeeding doesn't always happen. Some women have difficulty breastfeeding, others continue to eat like horses and you can't always be sure how Mother Nature will decide to dish out the hormones. Ultimately, you can't completely rely on breastfeeding to strip those kilos off.

Top Tips for Losing Baby Weight

Nutrition

- Eat well – eat when hungry and drink when thirsty, but no salty, sugary, fatty processed food. Eat for optimum nutrition. If you're breastfeeding, aim for an extra 200–500 calories a day, which should put you at around 1500–1800 calories per day.
- I'm not all that comfortable setting postnatal weight-loss targets, as the principle concern is your child. If you were overweight or obese *before* you fell pregnant, simply cleaning up the crap-food diet that got you there in the first place will see you shedding stacks of weight. If you gained a normal amount of weight during pregnancy (see the table on the previous page), you could aim to lose around half a kilogram a week, but don't forget to factor in an extra kilo of breast tissue into your weight-loss goals while you're feeding. And don't worry: losing 500 grams a week will not affect your milk production.

Exercise

- Start your exercise routine as soon as you feel ready to, but take it gently initially. Beginning at around six to eight weeks after childbirth is ideal.
- Walking is an excellent starting point, because you can take your baby with you and you can do it anywhere. Carry him or her in a sling, front pack or backpack – it's reassuring for your baby to be so close to you and the weight increases your load and calorie expenditure.
- Get yourself a good sports bra and try to exercise after breastfeeding, not before.
- Jogging strollers are excellent. You can run with friends or on your own, *and* spend time with your baby.
- I get lots of enquiries about getting rid of postnatal flabby tummies. Getting stored fat off this area is notoriously difficult, and getting stretched skin to look like it did before childbirth isn't any easier. Exercise, of course, is number one in my book. Not just abdominal exercises, although they won't always reinstate the muscles to their former glory, but exercise generally. It'll take time, but it'll happen.

> Michelle's program helped me rewire my brain so I could stop sabotaging myself with poor food choices and lack of motivation. I realised that diets don't work – this is a lifestyle change. I now feel I can do anything I put my mind to.

Jess, 26, Melbourne

My top 4 metabolism boosters

Now that you understand how a sluggish metabolism is a key reason why it's so hard to lose the last 5 kilos, I want to take you through my top 4 diet and exercise tips for **boosting** your metabolism.

1. Eat regularly

This is important. Your metabolism slows down when you sleep because **you are not eating** and cranks up again when you tuck into a good brekkie. Since your metabolism slows down without food, it makes sense to eat regularly during the day, **but what you eat is critical**. If your three meals are interspersed with crappy, high-calorie snacks like processed biscuits in a box with sloppy fake cheese, you will be defeating the purpose. Rather, see my snack suggestions on page 85.

Starting the day with a good breakfast also stops you playing games with yourself: 'If I skip breakfast and have an apple for lunch, I'm allowed to stuff myself when I get home.' Remember my mantra: 'Eat like a king for breakfast, a prince for lunch, and a pauper for dinner.' Take on board the calories when you need them and know how many calories you are consuming in a day!

2. Drink water

Apart from being an appetite suppressant, water is also essential for efficient kidney and liver function. These guys are responsible for breaking down and disposing of

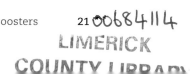

the waste products that you generate as you lose weight, so you need to keep both of them well hydrated. Not enough water? You slow the whole process down.

Water actually boosts your metabolism as your body has to expend energy warming it in your stomach so that it can be absorbed. But don't get too excited and start carrying around a thermos of iced spring water. Drinking a bottle of icy cold water only expends 25 calories, about the equivalent of either a carrot or a walnut.

How much water?

We're constantly told that we should drink eight glasses of water per day, but this is misleading. Does a 150 kilogram man need the same amount of water as a 55 kilogram woman? No. And besides, what's a glass? The truth is we need approximately 30 ml of water per kilo of body weight per day. An average tea cup holds 250 ml, and a water bottle 600 ml. I weigh 60 kilograms, so I'm going to need three bottles of water, or a couple of bottles of water and a couple of cups of tea per day to be roughly where I need to be.

3. Eat metabolism-boosting foods

Your body actually expends energy digesting, absorbing and storing food. This is referred to as the 'thermal effect' of food. Now, before you get too carried away with the notion of gorging yourself and shrinking away in the process, you need to be aware that the thermal effect of food accounts for only 5–10 per cent of your total daily calorie expenditure. By far the biggest calorie-burning factor is your basal metabolic rate (the energy required to keep your body functioning), which accounts for 65–75 per cent of your daily calorie expenditure. The remaining 15–30 per cent is accounted for by physical activity. Now that's not just going to the gym or going for a run. It's **all of your physical activity** – hanging out the washing, brushing your teeth, even scratching your bum.

Your body digests and metabolises different foods at different rates, and simple carbohydrates (including sugar and refined grains) are broken down the quickest. Protein is digested and metabolised the slowest, thereby expending the most energy. Fats are metabolised after carbs and before protein, and are converted directly to – you guessed it – fat.

Negative-calorie foods

There are some foods that actually have a **negative-calorie effect**. In other words, we actually expend more calories digesting and metabolising them than the number of calories they contain. This is because they are **hard** for your body to digest as they are fibrous and frequently eaten raw. Because they take longer to break down, they keep your metabolism fired up for longer. But that's not all: they're good for bowel health, are rich in nutrients, and also happen to be lowest in calories . . . do you see where this is going? Yep: the land of fruit and vegies.

Here are my favourites:

- **Vegetables**: lettuce, carrot, cucumber, broccoli, cauliflower, onion, radish, cabbage, asparagus, green beans, spinach, zucchini, beetroot, celery, garlic, turnip, chilli, watercress.
- **Fruits**: strawberry, apple, tomato, cranberry, mango, orange, pineapple, raspberry, tangerine, papaya, grapefruit, rockmelon (cantaloupe), watermelon, honeydew melon, blueberry, lemon, lime, peach.

Grains, vegetables, fruits and other fibrous foods are unrefined carbohydrates, and are digested slowly, keeping your insulin levels steady. This is important, because as we saw earlier, insulin is a hormone that tells your body to *store* fat.

Fish and seafood are really great choices, along with sea vegetables (kelp, seaweed) and shellfish. These foods are rich in iodine, which helps to keep your thyroid gland healthy. An under-active thyroid can lead to weight gain, depression and general bloody misery, so make sure there's iodine in your diet. If you're not keen on seafood it's also present in iodised salt (no surprise there), eggs and dairy products.

Fish has the added advantage of being a rich source of omega 3, an essential fatty acid (these are 'essential' because our bodies can't manufacture them, so we have to get them from our food). One of the groovy things that omega 3 does is to regulate a protein called leptin, which plays a major role in deciding whether your body will burn fat or store it. Now *that's* a protein that I want to take to lunch!

Low-fat yoghurt, milk and cheese are definitely on the menu because they're packed full of calcium, which can crank up your metabolism.

4. Balance strength and cardio training

Since we know that our metabolism slows down during sleep, it doesn't take a genius to work out that a training session first thing is a fantastic way to fire up the metabolism. If you're looking for a great workout, a killer calorie burn and more feel-good happiness than a gay dance party, you can't beat a solid 40-minute aerobic exercise session to get your heart rate up, and your waist measurement down. But, does it increase your metabolism? The short answer is yes, **but you will need to go hard** and it usually only lasts for as long as the session, tapering off quickly.

After exercise, our bodies need to get back to their normal resting state – a bit like cleaning up after a party. This includes building molecules and repairing cells, returning hormone levels to normal, developing our nervous system to accommodate any changes that have taken place, and relocating the free fatty acids in our bloodstream to name a few. All this takes energy, and that energy is sourced from increased oxygen intake **after you've finished training**. This 'after burn' is known as excess post-exercise oxygen consumption (EPOC) and can last anywhere from three to sixteen hours after your workout, depending on what kind of exercise you were doing, how hard you were doing it and how long you were doing it for.

Now, before you start bombarding me with emails wanting to know which exercises maximise after burn, I have to tell you that it's not 100 per cent clear. This is because it's difficult to compare the different types of exertion. However, I do know that although the EPOC effect is greater with weight training (anaerobic exercise), **aerobic exercise does use more calories during the session**.

You could argue that weight training has the added benefit of increasing your lean muscle mass, thereby increasing your metabolic rate, which would be true. But keep it real: 1 kilo of muscle will add 10–20 calories to your basal metabolic rate, and as any weight trainer will tell you, it takes a **lot of work to put on a kilo of muscle**. My philosophy is to do both! Aerobic or cardiovascular training coupled with weight training is the perfect combination for health, weight loss and weight management.

There is another excellent side effect of exercise: our muscles become more sensitive to insulin. This means that our body doesn't have to produce as much, and so there's less of it floating around in our bloodstreams. As we've seen, too much insulin in our bloodstream results in excessive conversion of sugar to fat. So exercise not only burns fat, but also helps to stop our bodies from making more insulin. Exercise rocks for *so* many reasons. You'd have to be outright bonkers not to do it!

Exercise also **lowers our levels of cortisol**. As we saw earlier, our adrenal gland pumps this stuff out by the bucket load during times of stress, and elevated levels of this 'flight or fight' hormone lead to (among other things) increased abdominal fat, the most dangerous fat repository of all. One of the reasons we feel so relaxed and chilled after a good workout is that there is less cortisol floating around our body, which in turn reduces fat deposits. Good, eh?

Since we know that our metabolism slows down during sleep, it doesn't take a genius to work out that a good training session first thing is a fantastic way to fire up the metabolism. You can't beat a solid 40-minute aerobic exercise session to get your heart rate up.

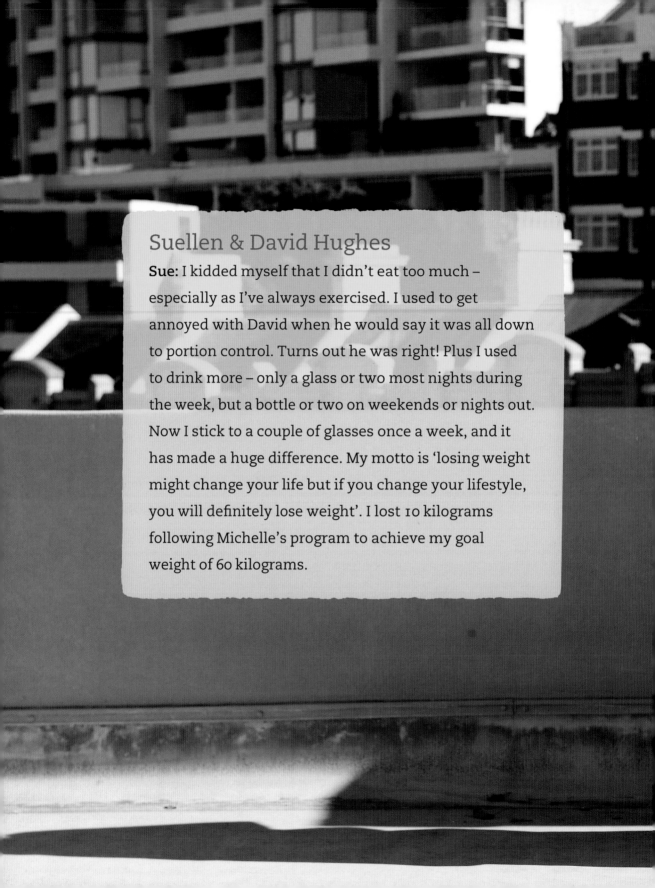

Suellen & David Hughes

Sue: I kidded myself that I didn't eat too much –
especially as I've always exercised. I used to get
annoyed with David when he would say it was all down
to portion control. Turns out he was right! Plus I used
to drink more – only a glass or two most nights during
the week, but a bottle or two on weekends or nights out.
Now I stick to a couple of glasses once a week, and it
has made a huge difference. My motto is 'losing weight
might change your life but if you change your lifestyle,
you will definitely lose weight'. I lost 10 kilograms
following Michelle's program to achieve my goal
weight of 60 kilograms.

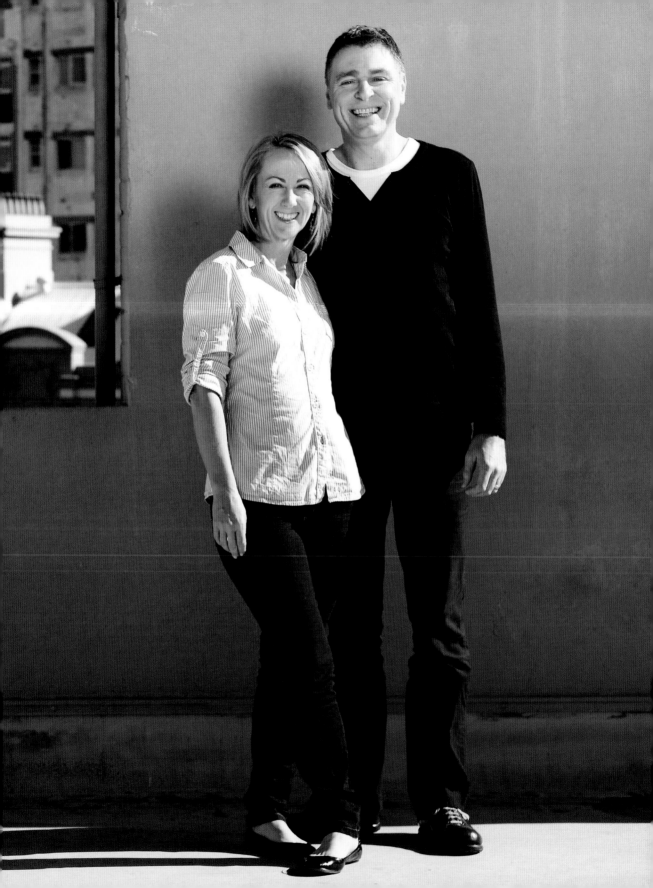

How our minds work against us

If you're only 5 kilos over your goal weight, you might think that tidying up your diet and boosting your exercise is all you'll need to do to reach your goal. But the truth is, **most of us already know this**, so there must be something missing from the equation. There is. It's the mind factor – the thoughts and feelings behind what we do (or don't do).

In *Crunch Time*, I talk about how crucial it is to examine your eating habits: to find out if there is a connection between what you eat and how you are feeling. Do you reach for a glass of wine (or five) when you are celebrating something? Do you hoe into a family block of chockie when you are feeling down or lonely? Do you use food as a reward for doing the housework or other chores, or to stave off boredom? Emotional eating is rampant (**all of my overweight or obese clients** are either emotional eaters, or have been at some stage of their lives) and many of us lapse in and out of this destructive eating pattern without even being aware of it. We often give children food to make them feel better and I believe this can be the beginning of a lifetime of emotional eating.

The excuses

Our bad habits (poor food choices, little exercise, emotional eating) thrive on a huge array of colourful excuses. Do you:

- Tell yourself you'll feel better if you eat something when you feel emotional, whether you are hungry or not?
- Find excuses for not exercising? (It's too cold/My ankle is sore)
- Find excuses for making poor food choices? (My children hate vegetables/I don't have anything in the fridge)

Excuses are basically of three types, and identifying their type is the first step to challenging them and coming up with new habits and behaviours.

> I knew Michelle's program was going to affect me physically (I have lost 43 kg since February 2010 and I'm fitter than I've ever been) but I was not prepared for what it's done for ME. To me. In me. In my mind, my heart, my thinking.

Jo, 33, Sydney

1. Internal excuses within your control

These are based around the old internal negotiation:

- 'I'm a bit tired tonight, so I won't train in case I hurt myself.'
- 'I've fallen off the wagon, so what's the point?'
- 'I'm not motivated. I'll wait and get a training partner to fire me up.'
- 'I am too unfit at the moment. I'll get myself back in shape then I'll go back to the gym' (I love that one!)

2. External excuses within your control

These are based around external factors over which you do have some control, but which you choose to allow to control you. For example:

- 'I'm really busy at work at the moment.'
- 'It's cold/wet outside and I might catch a cold.'
- 'It's too expensive at my local gym.'
- 'My training buddy can't make it tonight.'

3. External excuses out of your control

These are out-of-the-blue events that affect your training/nutrition such as a car accident, a sick child or a family crisis. Clearly you have no control over these situations, but once they have been resolved, make sure you get straight back into your training and healthy eating. When it comes to rocky times, I've found my training to be my saviour.

Once you work out the kind of excuses you're using to prevent yourself from eating right and training well, you can organise the mental ammo you will need to challenge them. Look at the example below and then draw up a list of your ten favourite excuses and your solutions.

Excuse	Type	Solution
'I'm really busy at work at the moment so I can't go to the gym.'	EXTERNAL	I'll organise my days so I *can* fit in my training. I deserve the break and I'll be more efficient and focused at work anyway.
'I'm a bit tired tonight, so I won't train in case I hurt myself.'	INTERNAL	I'll do it anyway. I'll get stronger so there's less chance of injury plus I'll sleep better.
'It's too cold/wet outside for training and I might catch a cold.'	EXTERNAL	I'll wear a hoodie, plus I'll soon warm up with exercise.
'I'll order take away tonight because I have nothing in the fridge.'	EXTERNAL	I know that I can stop at the grocer on my way home tonight and pick up what I need for a quick healthy meal.
'I'm not motivated. I'll wait until I get a training partner to fire me up.'	INTERNAL	I've got to learn to fly solo. The only way to do it is to do it. Consistency is the key, not motivation.
'It's too expensive at my local gym.'	EXTERNAL	I'll find another one near work, or start with running/cycling or some other training that doesn't cost money.
'I may as well eat whatever I want today because I'll start my eating plan on Monday.'	INTERNAL	This is the same old BS I've been dishing up to myself for years. It starts now with me saying NO and walking away.

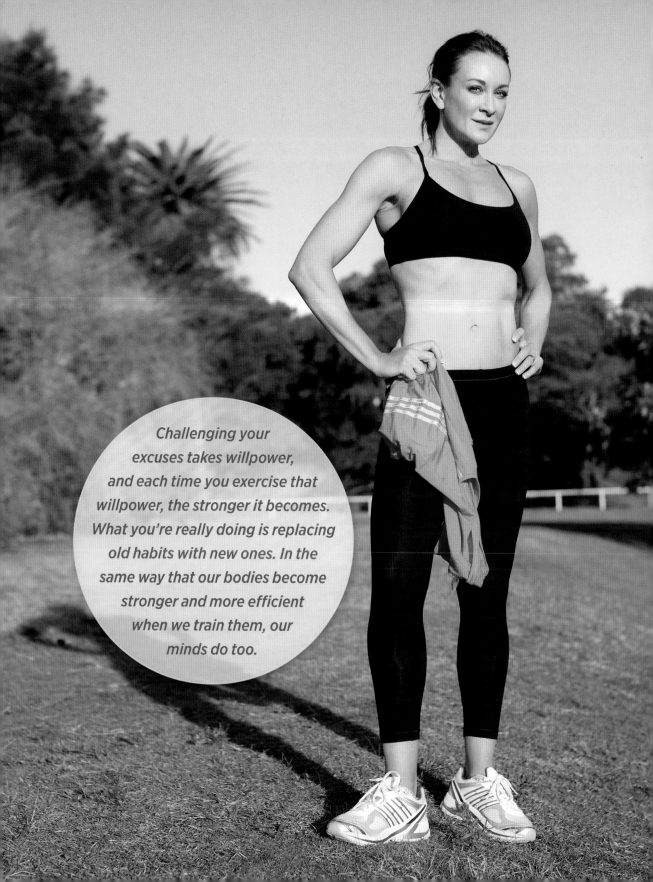

Challenging your excuses takes willpower, and each time you exercise that willpower, the stronger it becomes. What you're really doing is replacing old habits with new ones. In the same way that our bodies become stronger and more efficient when we train them, our minds do too.

Challenging your excuses takes willpower, and each time you exercise that willpower, the stronger it becomes. What you're really doing is replacing old habits with new ones. And don't give me any rubbish about how hard it is to learn new habits when you are older, either. That's just another excuse. Our brains are **wired for challenges** – they thrive on learning new stuff, and there's more and more research around to show that as we get older, we gotta use it or lose it. So keep coming up with alternatives.

One of my contestants told me about a brilliant method she used that she called the 'lay by' system or the 'cooling off' period. If she saw some chocolate she wanted to eat, she would 'put it on lay by' for twenty-four hours. If after twenty-four hours she still wanted it, she would eat it and then work it into her calorie count for the day. If she didn't want it, she'd just let it go.

By saying no the first time and walking away she was taking responsibility for her choice, and that was empowering. She wasn't telling herself that she **couldn't have the chocolate**, just that she would control **when she could have it**. But get this – saying no the first time made her resolve even stronger, so the next day she usually found herself saying no again. Cool, huh?

When you boil it all down, she had simply learned a new behaviour. How? She had first **changed the story she told herself**. Instead of saying 'I can't control myself – I just have to eat this now,' she said, 'I can choose when I eat this. I'm going to put this on lay by.'

> Before Michelle's program I was struggling, but it has given me not only the energy to live my life but a renewed sense of enthusiasm to be the best person I can be.

Kate, 27, Brisbane

Negative self-talk

To help you ditch your unhealthy habits around food and exercise, you'll also need to bust a few myths about yourself that you've been dragging around for years.

Stories like, 'I have the willpower of a labrador!' or 'I always end up chucking it in because I don't have any self-control.'

I believe in the power of language, so if you are saying these things out loud and in your head day in, day out, you are putting these negative messages out there to the universe big-time. If you say them, you believe them and you are **making them happen**.

The truth is that **none of these negative opinions is true**. Why? Because, you've almost always constructed these self-limiting thoughts in moments when emotion was running high and you weren't thinking clearly.

More than likely, you made a decision to go on a diet/health kick in the heat of the moment: after a fight, a binge, or after you spent three hours getting ready for an event which you didn't end up going to because you felt like a fat cow and so you burst into tears and consoled yourself with a family block of chocolate. Then, with the decision made to get stuck into a diet and exercise regime, you proceeded to go about it for approximately three or four days, after which time you kinda ran out of emotional steam and hey, it was your dad's birthday and you just felt too rude to say no to a piece of black forest cake.

Then, bang, you've proved to yourself once again that you have the willpower of an iceberg lettuce and you tell yourself that losing those last 5 kilos is forever out of your reach.

Right?

Wrong!

The problem is that you set your goal when you were feeling vulnerable and emotional. If you think about it, it's counterintuitive to expect ourselves to make **sound, logical decisions** when our prevailing mental state is charged with emotion.

One of the most common statements I hear from my weight-loss clients is that they have 'lost control' – and not just of their eating habits. They say they have lost control of their weight, their exercise patterns, and their lives in general. Later, when they've successfully regained their health and fitness, **they say the exact opposite**. 'I feel so much better in myself, so much more in control.' They are firmly planted in the driver's seat. These people haven't just exercised their bodies, they've also exercised their minds – when you get your head right, your body will follow

Mind training

In the same way that our bodies become stronger and more efficient when we train them, our minds do too. Here are ten 'exercises' in mind fitness that you can use daily. Some are based on your approach to physical training, others on nutrition and a couple are based on everyday life. Of course, following the 30-day workout and menu plan in this book will sharpen your **mind and body fitness** in ways you never thought possible, however, you might find a couple of these exercises an interesting way to test your preparedness to go the whole hog on the 30-day plan.

Ten exercises for mind fitness

1. Instead of coming home from work and sitting on your butt, pick yourself up, put on your runners and get out the door.
2. If you drink coffee, go a whole week without sugar and make it skim milk; plus, if you usually have two or three coffees a day, knock it down to one and savour it!
3. Walk, run or cycle all or part of the way to work twice a week.
4. Take the stairs every chance you get for one week. If you don't know where they are, find them, even if they are the fire stairs.
5. Next weekend, offer to do the gardening for someone you care about (wife, husband, partner, parents or friend, etc).
6. Choose to drink water rather than alcohol at a weekend social event.
7. Pick one chore that has been hanging over your head for months and do it.
8. Go for one week without any chocolate.
9. Hold your tongue when you catch yourself about to pass judgement on someone or something.
10. Choose two nights in a week where you don't watch any TV and you go for a walk instead.

I am halfway to my goal and KNOW I will get there. I am so happy and confident now. My energy is amazing. I love training and my family love the healthy, yummy recipes. They especially love the happy healthy me. So much energy, a new lease on life. My results have far exceeded my expectations.

Amanda, 41, Sydney

Everyone can do these exercises – you don't need to spend a lot of money or organise any special equipment. Just do them with integrity and feel your sense of empowerment grow!

Consistency vs. motivation

Of all the questions that I am asked about exercise and healthy living (and God knows there are plenty to choose from: what to eat, when to train, should I stretch, whether to do weights or cardio), there is one that endlessly haunts me: 'So tell me, Michelle, how do you stay motivated?' When I hear it, I want to tear my hair out, because what I do is not about motivation, it's about consistency. **Motivation is about feeling** – determined, enthusiastic, frenzied, angry – and is therefore fickle and unreliable like a bad ex-boyfriend. You can't count on it being there because we know feelings or emotions do not last, and if your journey is based on feeling motivated it won't last either. Consistency, however, **is about doing**. Consistency isn't something that you need to wind up like a coiled spring every morning. You don't need to plug it in and re-charge it every few hours. It is that steady, yet relentless, journey to an end. It doesn't require profound thought. You quite literally **just do it**. In fact I have a T-shirt that makes the point a little more emphatically by boasting my favourite acronym on the front in bold letters: 'J F D I'.

When I've racked up a fifteen-hour day and I'm driving past the gym on the way home, **do I feel motivated**? When my alarm goes off at 5 a.m. and it's seven degrees and raining outside, **do I feel motivated**? Are you nuts? Sure – motivated to **stay in bed**!

So here are my tips for consistency:

1. **Don't think, just do**. Just put on your gym gear, head out the door and get over it.

2. Don't start bargaining with yourself. No trade-offs – none of that 'maybe I could skip this morning and go for a run at lunch time' bullshit. **Just get on with it**.

3. If you feel yourself wavering, apply the Ten Minute Rule. Start your workout and train for just ten minutes. If you still don't feel like it after ten minutes, then treat yourself to going back to bed and a lie in. Trust me – it doesn't happen. In fact, some of my best workouts have come off the back of a Ten Minute Ruler.

I once had an obese client whose doctor would not allow him to elevate his heart rate above 100 beats per minute. Basically all he could do was walk. Plus he was only allowed to walk for thirty minutes at a time, three times a day. The guy was forty-eight years of age and obese – classic heart-attack material. I decreased his calories to 1300 a day – which was pretty much all I could do. He stuck to his menu plan and did his ninety minutes of walking and **he lost an amazing 10 kilos** in the first week! In his case it wasn't about intensity, but consistency. And we all have the power of consistency. Think about it – we have consistently gone back for seconds, consistently gone to yum cha on Sundays, consistently bought a chocolate bar when filling up at the servo and consistently got a headache whenever anyone ever suggests going for a walk. We're fantastic at it! Now it's just a matter of being consistent with the right habits.

If you want to know my recipe for success, just read the T-shirt!

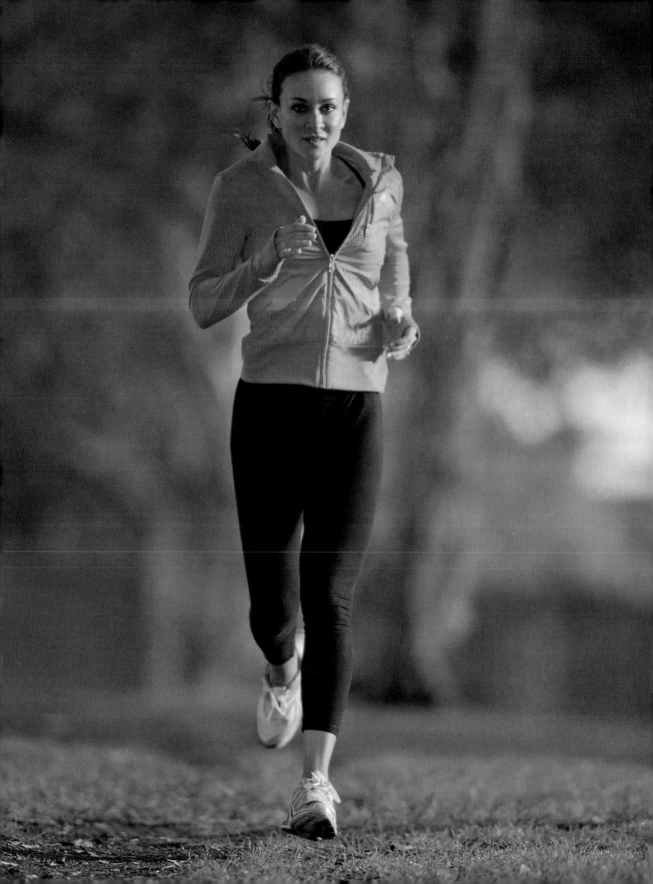

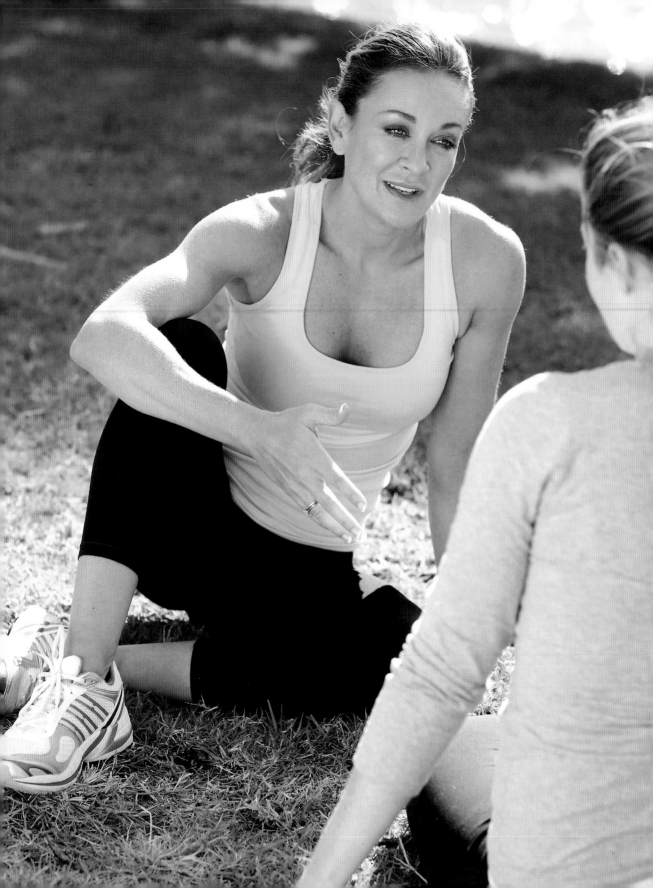

how to do it

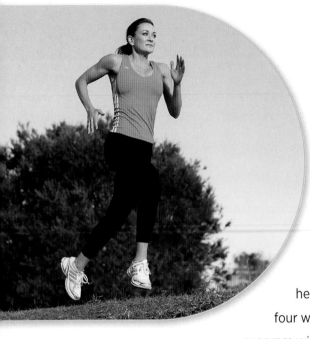

My 30-day menu & workout plan

NOW THAT YOU UNDERSTAND why it's been so tough to lose those last 5 kilos, you're in the right head space to take on my 30-day plan. For the next four weeks you will be on a mission. Your weekly training program will consist of three fitness days, two strength/cardio days and one light fitness and core strength day. Yep, it'll be six days a week for the next four weeks. I've kept the exercises simple so you can do them at a gym or at home (if you have the space and a minimum of equipment). I've also included a fitness test, which will set the benchmark. We will revisit the test at the halfway mark and again at the end of the 30 days in order to gauge your progress. Remember, this program is not only about losing weight, it's also about getting fit and strong.

The menu plan has 1200 total calories per day for women and 1800 for men. For women, each meal has around 300 to 350 calories and each snack is between 100 and 150 calories. For men each meal has around 450 calories (add a bit more lean protein – meat or fish) and each snack is about 200 calories. It's as simple as that. I've kept the easier recipes for the weekdays and the fancier ones for the weekend, when you'll have more time. You'll find my snacks suggestions on page 85 but feel free to come up with your own – as long as they stay within your calorie quota. Remember to keep your fruit snacks for mornings and vegetable snacks for the afternoons.

Here's what you need to do before we get started. These are absolutely non-negotiable – skip these tasks and the 30-day plan will not work. And remember, no alcohol for the next 30 days. Let's get it happening!

Organise your training locations

Health club/gym

Gyms are great because you can train in all weathers. You can often get a really good deal for a one-month membership and you can sometimes negotiate with them to waive the joining fee. Ask for a free personal training session if it's not already part of the membership package. Then, show the trainer this program and get them to run you through all the equipment to help you get started.

Outdoors

Training outside is fun, super convenient and cheap! There is plenty of running in my 30-day program, especially the fitness test, so you will need to find a running/walking route which you can use for 30-minute and 1-hour sessions. An athletics oval is great as it usually has a 400-metre circumference. If you can drive your running route you can use your car's odometer to get the distances.

For outdoor sessions you'll also need:

- Some benches
- Some steps at about knee-height and lower
- A set of stairs
- A clear grassy area where you can set up your circuits

Training backup plan

If you can't do one of your training sessions outdoors or at a gym, a cardio and strength DVD is a great backup. I recommend my *Seek & Destroy Cardio Kicker*, *Super Shredder Circuit* and *Tight Toned Terrific* because they cover both fitness and strength exercises in both high- and low-impact versions. (I've had a 70-year-old woman doing *Seek & Destroy*, so you'll be fine!)

I had never run in my life before February this year. Since then I've done a mini-triathalon in the gym and finished the City 2 Surf. My daughter thinks I rock!

Elizabeth, 56, Adelaide

Indoors

If you're super busy, then working out indoors is about as convenient as it gets! You will need a few things to set yourself up, though. An area where you can train unimpeded (a lounge room, spare room or similar) is important and you'll need some basic equipment, which you can buy from any sports or department store:

- A set of dumbbells 3–6 kilograms or heavier, depending on how strong you are
- A step, either in your house or an adjustable, portable one
- A fitball
- A barbell.

Training gear

- A good pair of runners.
- A comfortable, good-quality fitness outfit (T-shirt or tank top, bottoms and a long-sleeved top). Two sets is good so that you can have one in the wash. Taking some pride in your workout gear helps you feel the part and boosts your self-image when running or exercising outdoors or in the gym.
- Women need a good sports bra.
- A heart-rate monitor is incredibly useful as it helps you understand the relationship between your heart rate, your exercise and how many calories you are burning. Everyone who gets one says they suddenly understand why their training never worked before. It's not compulsory, but I rate them.
- Music is not essential, but it can keep you going when you think you just can't take another step.

Take your measurements

Jump on the **scales**, first thing in the morning, totally starkers and after you've been to the loo. You will be weighing in once a week at the start of each week in the same way, so always use the same scales.

Grab a **tape measure** and measure yourself as I've outlined below. We will also be doing this weekly, so wear the same clothes. I recommend firm-fitting clothes or just go nude!

- Chest: align the tape with your nipples.
- Waist: align the tape with your belly button.
- Hips: measure at your widest point.
- Thigh: place your foot on a low step (always use the same step), loop the tape around your thigh and slide it forwards and back until you find the widest point. Record your measurement, but also mark the point with a pen and then measure how far it is from the very tip of your kneecap. Next time you measure your thigh, you'll first find the kneecap-thigh point so that you're measuring at the same position.

If you think about your past attempts at shifting the last 5 kilos, I'll put money on the fact that you came unstuck when an unknown variable pulled you off track because you were disorganised. Schedule your training and plan your shopping, cooking and meals.

Lastly, take a **photo** of yourself in your underwear or swimmers. I know I'm really pushing the friendship here, but you'll be *so* glad you did this when you reach your goal.

Mark up your diary/calendar

Okay, this step is powerful! This is where you set yourself up for success! If you think about your past attempts at shifting the last 5 kilos, I'll put money on the fact that you came unstuck when an unknown variable pulled you off track because **you were disorganised**. To stop this happening again, you will need to not only schedule your training but also plan your grocery shopping, cooking and meals.

Schedule in your training

First mark in your diary (or on your calendar) the day you will do your first Fitness Test. Then schedule in your training sessions, including what they will be and where and when you'll be doing them. I strongly recommend early-morning training as it's a great way to start the day, the monkey is off your back and you are less likely to be disrupted by your work or your family.

This is how your training will be set up:

MONDAY DAY 1: fitness

TUESDAY DAY 2: strength/toning

WEDNESDAY DAY 3: fitness

THURSDAY DAY 4: strength/toning

FRIDAY DAY 5: light fitness /core strength /stretch

SATURDAY DAY 6: super fitness day

SUNDAY DAY 7: rest

Each night, make sure you're on top of what is happening for your training the next morning. Have your group fitness timetable handy, get your clothes out, check the weather conditions and have a back-up plan.

Mark in all your 'red flag' days – the social events, birthdays, holidays, work functions, interstate travel and school holidays that you'll need to work around. Red flag days are super important because these are when most people fall off the wagon.

Schedule in your shopping and cooking

Try to do your 'big shop' on the same day each week, like a Thursday night, and work out which day will be convenient to do a 'top-up' shop. I provide shopping lists, so there's no excuse for not having the right ingredients!

Plan your cooking days and when you might make extra portions for lunch the next day or freeze for another dinner later in the week. I like to cook up extras at night for the following day and I also cook up a big soup or stew on Sunday, put it in meal size portions in containers, and freeze it for the week.

Tell people who care

This is where you now make your commitment out loud. This is about putting yourself at the top of the priority list and giving yourself as much time as you give others. (If this makes you uncomfortable, think about the fact that by giving to yourself, you will be able to give so much more to others anyway.)

Start by writing, 'My commitment is to lose 5 kilos in one month (plus any other goals you have set yourself, e.g. 'fit into my favourite black dress', 'try rock-climbing', 'go swimming in public') and I am prepared to do the work it takes to get there'. Stick this up somewhere you can see it daily.

Now, call a family meeting and make sure you have everyone's full attention (no radios, TVs, electronic devices). Be open and heartfelt about your goals for self-improvement, and how important it is that you achieve them. Although you don't need your family's approval and support to do this, it really is very helpful on a practical level if you have it. You need to explain that you will be eating differently and that as a family you will all be taking better care of your health and nutrition. Junk food will no longer be freely available. If and when the complaints start, remember that **you are the main role model** in your children's lives – showing them how to look after their nutrition is one of the greatest gifts you can give them.

Then share your goal with your friends. Call them, drop in and say hi or enter it on your Facebook page.

Michelle's program is like nothing else. It's as though there was one single piece of information that my brain needed to figure out to understand what losing weight was all about – and I sure found it.

Amanda, 41, Sydney

Case study

At 36, Meghan was a relatively active person. She worked part time, walked twice a week, did a Pilates class every now and then and was busy running a house and a family. But since the birth of her children, she hadn't paid much attention to her health and fitness and felt that it was starting to show.

Meghan's energy levels were low, she didn't sleep well and her self-confidence had waned. She avoided undressing in front of a mirror (or her husband), chose to be the photographer rather than be in the picture and wore more loose-fitting clothing.

Meghan had exercised fairly regularly when she was younger, and played team sport at school. She'd dabbled in swimming and tennis once she started work, but that had fallen by the wayside as the years passed and marriage and children took priority. Meghan felt unfit and was definitely sitting about 8 kilograms over her ideal weight.

At 163 centimetres and 68 kilograms, she was at the low end of the 'overweight' category on the body mass index (BMI) chart. The problem was that as she moved into her forties, a further decline in her fitness guaranteed further weight gain and its attendant health issues.

Meghan decided to change her future.

She became a client of mine, and as with all my new clients, I was very straight with Meghan from the onset. I asked her what she expected to achieve and told her what she needed to do to get there. Meghan was very clear about what she wanted and quite adamant that she was prepared to do the work to get there. Cool!

The plan was for her to get from 68 to 62 kilograms. We set up an exercise and eating plan for her to lose 6 kilograms in six to eight weeks. Before training started, I had Meghan go through her diary to make the time for six training sessions a week. She would see me once a week and the rest of the sessions were made up of classes and cardio and weight training programs at the gym.

Meghan had chosen to exercise in the mornings when she could pop her youngest child into the gym's crèche. On the days she worked, she got up early to train and hubby would get the kids up. On Saturday she and her husband took turns training so one of them was always at home to care for the children. Importantly, I made her go through her diary for the next eight weeks and circle all her 'red flag' days: birthdays, social events, family get-togethers, etc. I asked her to plan ahead for her training on these days, and to be prepared to meet the food challenges that these events usually present.

Next was the kitchen clean-out. All the foods that were holding her back were gone. I think this step was more confronting than Meghan had expected, as she later confided in me that she found it really difficult to throw food away, even if it had zero nutritional value. Meghan was also in shock when she stepped back and considered some of the food she was feeding her family. Already she was starting to battle some demons!

Although Meghan was not a big drinker, she had a glass of wine, sometimes two, with her husband most nights. I asked Meghan if she was willing to give up alcohol six days out of seven, and she agreed.

Now we were ready to start. I took all her measurements, weighed her in and training began. In the first week she lost 2.3 kilograms! Amazing! She turned up for every training session (and really went for it in most of them), cleaned out her diet and upped her incidental activity (e.g. taking the stairs and walking whenever possible). She was pumped! This was her best result in all of the weeks we trained together, but that was enough to spur her on. By the fourth week she'd lost 5.2 kilograms, 800 grams short of her 6 kilogram goal!

Meghan went on to lose a further 2.5 kilograms over the next four weeks, which put her at 60.5 kilograms, giving her a total of 7.7 kilograms in eight weeks. Not bad! Besides that, she had become quite fit and had set herself a new goal in the fourth week: to run/walk a half marathon in a month's time. Meghan's husband also lost a staggering 10 kilograms in the same time frame by going for a run in his lunch hour and following the same meal plan.

Here was this ordinary couple doing extraordinary things. They were energised now, and were looking to do new things together as a family, like bike riding on the weekends. They also agreed that they both felt sexier.

Now, several years later, I still see Meghan down at the gym doing her morning training. Last time we spoke both she and her husband had just completed a mini triathlon. She was rapt! When I asked her what her time was she said, 'I don't really know or care. I'm still smiling about the fact that I was out there in my cossie in *public* and I loved it!'

In week four of Michelle's program I was rock climbing. In week seven I ran 7 kms. I increased my swimming distance from 200 metres to 1000 metres.

Kathy, 64, Melbourne

Clean up your kitchen

Your nutrition is **EVERYTHING!** In order for you to drop those last 5 kilos you are going to have to clean out all the crap food which has been holding you back, and restocking your pantry and fridge with food which will get you lean and mean fast! And for the next month you won't be drinking alcohol either, so give it to friends or store it in the cellar and forget about it.

Drag your wheelie bin close to the back door and start chucking! Be ruthless. Soft drinks, lollies, biscuits, potato chips, sugary breakfast cereals and processed crap have **got to go**. Don't even think about it being a 'waste'. It's not even food, and shouldn't be fed to anyone in your family! The real 'waste' is all these years that you've felt miserable about your weight, fitness and health.

Food to toss

- Processed cereals: check the nutritional panels because often the ones you think are 'healthy' are not. Breakfast cereals should have a maximum of 1.5 grams of fat and 200 calories per serve (excluding milk)
- Processed snacks: biscuits, chips, rollups, salty nuts, muesli bars, chocolate, lollies, fatty dips
- Cakes, biscuits, packet muffins, pancake mixes
- Frozen packet food (e.g. puff pastry, pies, fish fingers, nuggets)
- White bread, two-minute noodles
- Sugary and salty spreads and condiments (e.g. jam, tomato sauce)
- Cream, high-fat cheese (e.g. cream cheese, brie), ice cream
- Soft drink, cordial and processed juice.

Food essentials

I won't go into too much detail here as each week I'll give you a specific shopping list to cover you for the week, but here's a rough guide to what you'll need in the pantry, fridge or freezer:

- Milk, low-fat/low-cal or soy
- Cottage cheese
- Garlic (fresh)
- Ginger (fresh)
- Onions
- Eggs
- Flour, buckwheat and wholemeal self-raising
- Sugar, brown
- Bread: flat wholemeal/mountain, rye or wholegrain
- Muesli, untoasted
- Rolled oats
- Special K
- Quinoa
- Couscous
- Brown rice
- Wheat, cracked
- Soba noodles
- Lentils, French-style green
- Cans of: beans (butter, chickpeas, red kidney), tomatoes, tuna, salmon, sardines, baby beetroot
- Broad beans, frozen
- Mustard, wholegrain

- Dried herbs and spices: chilli, coriander, cumin, dukkah, paprika, saffron, spice mixes (Cajun and ras el hanout), turmeric
- Olive oil and olive oil spray
- Peppercorns, whole black
- Sesame seeds
- Stock, vegetable, salt-reduced
- Fish sauce
- Oyster sauce
- Soy sauce, salt-reduced
- Vinegar for dressings (red-wine, white-wine, balsamic)
- Tomato paste
- Anchovies
- Capers
- Nuts: almonds, walnuts
- Cranberries, dried
- Raisins

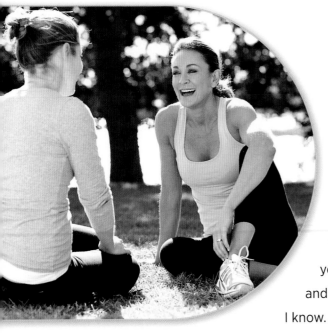

the fitness test

YOU NEED TO DO THIS FITNESS TEST BEFORE you start my program, at the end of week two and at the end of week four – three times in total. I know. Say the word 'test' and everybody freaks out. Relax. You will be fine. Every time I do a fitness test with my clients they are always a bit unsure to start with, but in the end they're very glad to be able to compare their results as the weeks pass and they get fitter! It's a great way to stay inspired.

This first test is simply a benchmark we can use to see how much fitter and stronger you've become. In other words, don't stress about what you get or don't get in the first test. The real fun begins when you re-test. That's when you get to see the results.

What you need

- A stopwatch or timer
- A 1-kilometre training route. It's best to use a standard athletics oval – two and a half laps equals 1 kilometre. Always use the same oval for all your testing. If there isn't one nearby, use the odometer of your car to find an exact 1-kilometre route. I would prefer you not to use a treadmill as it sets the pace and this test needs to be done under your own steam!

- A wall to lean against
- A place for push-ups and sit-ups
- A bench for triceps dips
- A page of your journal titled, 'Fitness Test Results'.

Before you do your fitness test you will need to spend about ten minutes warming up with a light jog and some basic stretching (see page 160). Make sure you stretch out your hamstrings, calves, chest, shoulders and triceps.

> *The hardest style of training for me is the intervals (running). They really scared the life out of me at the beginning (and I LOVE running), but they sure do produce results, so they have quickly turned into my favourite.*

Kate, 27, Brisbane

1. Cardio test: 1 kilometre time trial

This is designed to measure your cardiovascular fitness (basically how efficiently your heart pumps oxygen around your body). Use the oval, standard athletics track or street route that you have selected. Do your best, but I honestly don't care if you run, walk or crawl, **just get it done!** And don't forget to time yourself!

If you absolutely *cannot* do this for whatever reason (e.g. severe ankle injury or some other disability), then a 500-metre sprint on a rowing machine will suffice, but again time yourself.

Now record your time on your 'Fitness Test Results' page (see page 56).

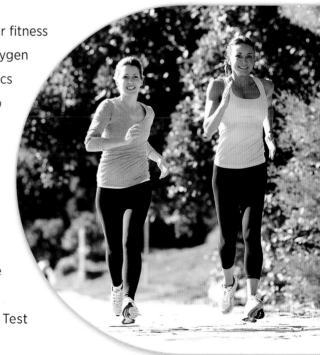

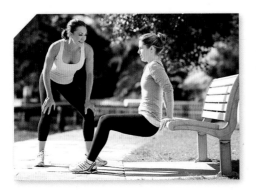

2. Upper-body strength tests: push-ups and triceps dips

This test will measure your upper-body strength and endurance and is divided into two parts. First you'll count how many push-ups you can do in 1 minute, and then how many triceps dips in a minute.

For the **push-ups**, your hands need to be slightly wider than shoulder-width apart, your spine long, neck extended, shoulders away from ears, and your abs pulled in. Your body should feel like a 'plank'. Girls can do these on their knees, and boys can choose. I would like everyone to eventually have a go at knocking out a couple on the toes. A proper push-up means you will need to get down to approximately 8 centimetres off the ground, so no cheating!

Now record your time on your 'Fitness Test Results' page.

For the **triceps dips**, start by sitting on a bench, hands palms down beside your hips, the heel of the hand on the edge of the bench. Take your body weight off the bench with your legs bent to approximately 90 degrees. Keep your butt close to the bench as if you are about to scratch your back, your chest proud, shoulders back and down, neck long, chin pulled in and eyes looking straight ahead. Try to have your arm bent at close to a right angle.

Now record your time on your 'Fitness Test Results' page.

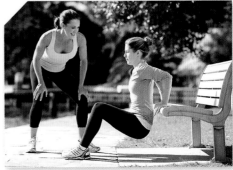

3. Lower-body strength test: the wall sit

The idea is to find out how long you can hold this position perfectly still.

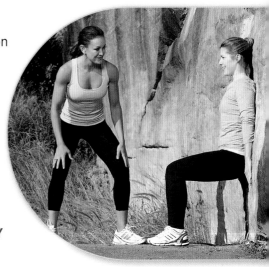

Position yourself against a solid wall, sliding down it until you are in a 'sitting' position. Your knees should be at right angles, hips level, abs pulled in, chest proud, back pressed against the wall, shoulder back and down, head against the wall. If you're holding the stop watch, start it now. If someone is helping, get them to start it.

When you can no longer hold that position **PERFECTLY STILL**, stop the watch.

Record your time on your 'Fitness Test Results' page.

4. Abdominal/core strength test: five-level sit-ups

We used this test in *The Biggest Loser Master Class* and it works a treat. It's a five-stage abdominal strength test where you move to the next stage if you successfully complete the previous stage. The rules are that your heels MUST stay on the ground. If they do, you can move to the next level. You only have to complete one sit-up at whichever level you make it to. Record your level on 'Fitness Test Results' page.

Level 1 – Wrists to kneecaps.

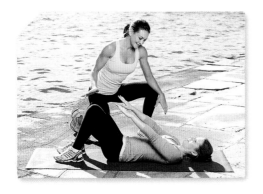 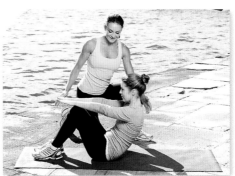

Level 2 – Arms across chest, full sit-up with elbows touching thighs.

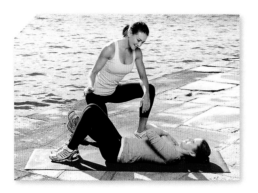 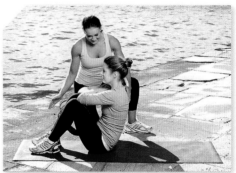

Level 3 – Hands linked behind head, elbows must remain out wide, full sit-up.

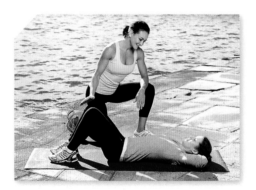 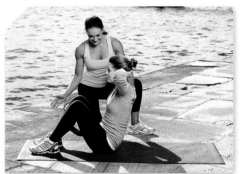

Level 4 – Arms crossed behind your head, fingers touching opposite shoulders, full sit-up.

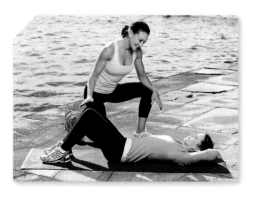 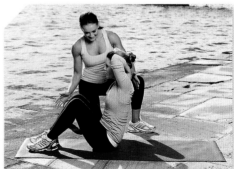

Level 5 – Arms fully extended and crossed behind head, full sit-up.

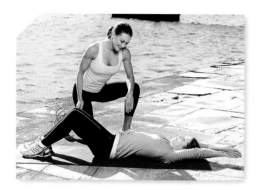 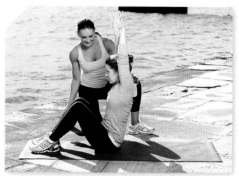

Record your results on your 'Fitness Test Results' page.

5. *Flexibility test*

Flexibility is often overlooked in fitness assessments. This test measures the flexibility of your hamstrings (backs of your legs) and lower back.

Sit on the ground, keeping your legs straight (calves and hamstrings touching the floor), stretch your arms straight forward with your hands flat on top of one another.

Have someone measure the distance from the tip of your shoes to your fingertips using a ruler or a builder's retractable measuring tape. Low flexibility means you will be a fair way short of reaching your toes. If you are super flexible you will be able to reach past your toes. Give yourself three chances and go with the best result.

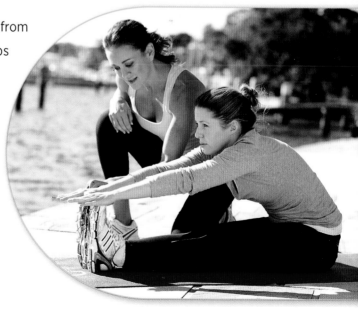

Record your measurements on your 'Fitness Test Results' page.

Fitness Test Results

Just as the scales talk to you about your weight loss, the fitness test talks to you about your fitness gain! This is an essential tool in measuring your success in the 30-Day Plan so make sure you record your results accurately before you start, at the halfway mark and finally at the end of the four weeks. You'll be amazed at your own progress!

		before you start	end of week 2	the finish line
1. Cardio test				
2. Upper-body strength tests	Push-ups			
	Triceps dips			
3. Lower body strength test				
4. Abdominal/core strength test				
5. Flexibility test				

Accelerator days

An 'accelerator day' (an expression first coined by my mate Andrew Simmons) is basically one day in a week where you remove most of your carbohydrates (such as oats, cereals, bread, rice, pasta, fruit, and heavier vegetables like sweet potatoes), but still train as you normally would. It is **not meant to be something** you do long term – it is a short-term proposition only, as in one day. It's similar to what a boxer or a jockey might do to shred an extra kilo in preparation for a specific event.

The first time I use accelerator days with clients I usually make it on a Sunday or on a day when they don't train, then later move it to a normal training day so that they really churn through the calories. While accelerator days don't work for everyone (some get good results and others show no benefit at all), they have worked for me personally and for many of my clients on my Twelve-Week Body Transformation Program (www.12wbt.com).

Since this is a short-term program and we're trying to get maximum results in a short period of time, you will be doing an accelerator day once a week on Tuesdays, with a 1200-calorie maximum for girls and a 1800-calorie max for guys. I've chosen Tuesdays because they feature strength and toning exercises, which are not as strenuous as cardio days. Friday might appear to be the obvious choice because it's a light training day, but because you have your 'super fitness day' on Saturday, you'll need some petrol in the tank to get you through the workouts.

Maureen Crook

After losing 30-odd kilograms to get from 95 to 65 kilograms, I still felt I had weight to lose. I tried more exercise, then I tried to diet, but nothing seemed to work for me. Michelle's exercise program was like having a personal trainer 24 hours a day. If I missed a gym class I could use the gym machines, or even workout in the local park (which I really enjoyed). And I loved having a ready-made menu that took the guesswork out of dinner. Not only did I get to my goal weight of 60 kilograms, but I now weigh 58! I feel fantastic and am so happy with myself!

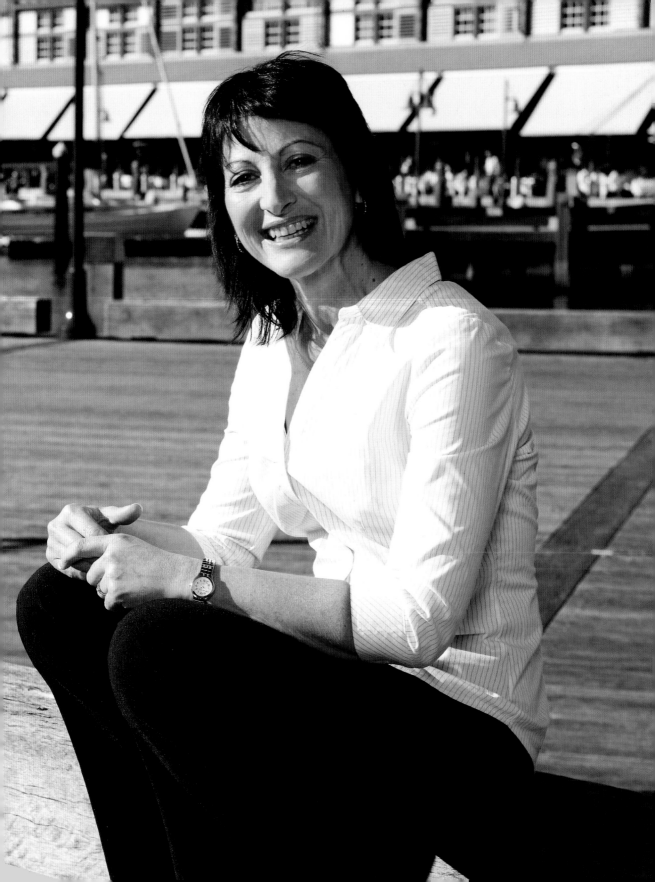

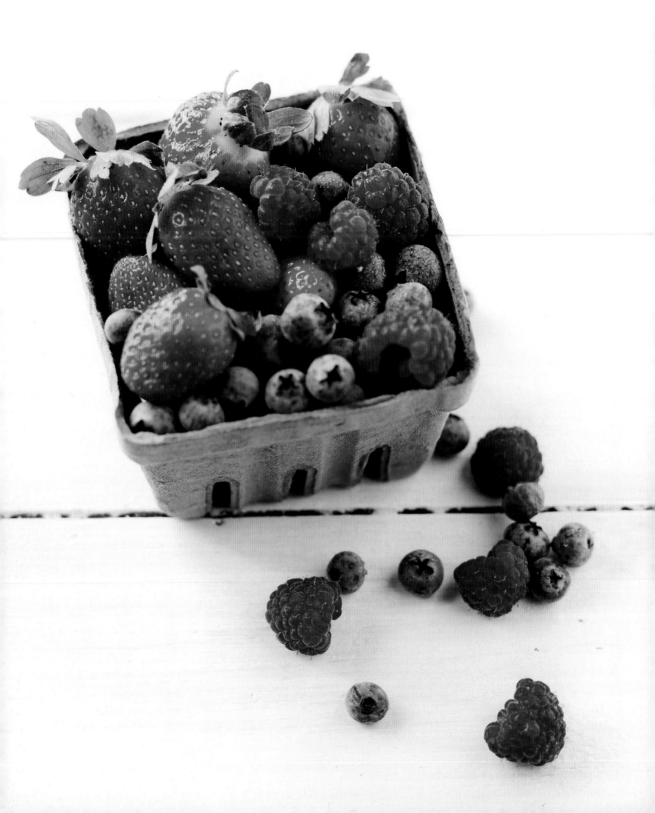

week 1

Be true to your word. Now is the time for integrity, self-respect and commitment.

Here we go! Week 1 is an opportunity for you to prove to yourself just what you can do with your health, fitness and weight. I am really excited for you!

Right from the start I ask for your commitment. What is the commitment you are making to your family, your friends, to me and more importantly to yourself? Are you a man or woman of your word?

You are worthy. You are amazing. And you are about to find out just how much!

My commitment is _____

shopping list and menu plan

Asparagus

Avocados

Bananas

Basil

Beef fillets

Berries, fresh, mixed

Blueberries

Bok Choy, baby

Bream, whole

Broccolini

Capsicums, green

Capsicums, red

Capsicums, yellow

Carrots, baby

Carrots

Cauliflower

Celeriac

Celery

Chicken breast fillets

Chillies, long red

Coriander

Corn on the cob

Cottage cheese

Cucumbers, Lebanese

Dill

Eggplant

Endive, curly

Fetta, low-fat/lo-cal

Garlic chives

Lemons

Lentils, French-style
   green

Limes

Mint

Mushrooms, field

Mushrooms, shiitake

Octopus, baby

Oregano

Parsley

Prawns, raw, medium

Ricotta, low-fat/lo-cal

Rocket

Shallots

Smoked salmon

Snapper fillets

Spinach, baby

Spinach, English

Strawberries

Tomatoes

Tomatoes, baby roma

Tomatoes, cherry

Tomatoes, roma

Tuna fillets

Wombok

Yoghurt, plain,
   low-fat/lo-cal

Yoghurt, vanilla,
   low-fat/lo-cal

Zucchinis

Remember, men can add a little more protein to each meal to make a total of 1800 calories per day, including snacks. Women: 1200 calories per day!

	breakfast	lunch	dinner	total cals
monday STIRFRY NIGHT	Quinoa porridge with cranberries and raisins 331 cal	Smoked salmon and salad wrap 302 cal	Stir-fried snapper with asparagus, wombok and shiitake mushrooms 260 cal	**893** **+ 307** *cal for snacks*
tuesday ACCELERATOR DAY!	Four egg-white omelette 300 cal	Pepper-crusted tuna with curly endive and cherry tomatoes 291 cal	Pan-fried chicken with steamed Asian greens (make more of the chicken for lunch tomorrow) 303 cal	**894** **+ 306** *cal for snacks (vegies only)*
wednesday WEIGH-IN DAY!	Quinoa porridge with cranberries and raisins 331 cal	Chicken wrap **or** Cucumber, beetroot, chicken and mint salad (using extra chicken from last night's dinner) 259 cal	Chermoula prawn kebabs with couscous 301 cal	**891** **+ 309** *cal for snacks*
thursday	Boiled egg and soldiers 295 cal	Smoked salmon and salad wrap **or** Lentil salad with yellow capsicum, coriander and cranberries 302 cal	Beef fillet with coriander salsa (make extra beef to pop into a sandwich for lunch tomorrow) 302 cal	**899** **+ 301** *cal for snacks*
friday CURRY NIGHT	Quinoa porridge with cranberries and raisins 331 cal	Beef or tuna and salad sandwich (using the leftovers from the beef last night) 300 cal	Cauliflower and celeriac Madras curry (make plenty of this and freeze in portions for next week's dinners or lunches) 269 cal	**900** **+ 300** *cal for snacks*
saturday	Fluffy buckwheat pancakes with berries and yoghurt 329 cal	Thai octopus salad 247 cal	Oven-baked whole bream with garlic spinach 299 cal	**875** **+ 325** *cal for snacks*
sunday	Pan-fried field mushrooms and tomatoes with fetta and oregano 310 cal	Spiced chargrilled vegetables with minted cracked wheat (make up extra portions of this for Monday lunch or dinner) 281 cal	Steamed minted chicken with broccolini and baby carrots (make up extra chicken for lunches during the week) 279 cal	**870** **+ 330** *cal for snacks*

workout program

Day 1: monday: **fitness/cardio**

CLASS Body Attack, Spin, Boxing, Cardio Circuit, Dance **or**
CIRCUIT ↓ Perform twice through, with a 1½-min rest between each round.

- Two laps of 400m oval *or* 800m treadmill run *or* 4 min park run
- 16 × jumping jacks
- 16 × triceps dips off a bench
- 16 × mountain climbers
- 16 × fast low-step running right leg
- 16 × push-ups (knees or toes)
- 16 × fast low-step running left leg

HERO MOMENT one sprint around 400m oval *or* run the full length around your park. Time yourself.

ABS Do 16 reps of each exercise, the whole set 3 times through.
- crunches
- twisting crunch to right
- twisting crunch to left

Day 2: tuesday: **toning/strength** *accelerator day*

CLASS Body Pump, strength/weights-based class **or**
SUPER SETS ↓ Do 16 reps of each exercise, and perform each 'super' set 3 times through before moving on to the next one (there are three super sets in all). The idea is to work with a strong technique and also with a sense of urgency. Keep recoveries to a minimum in order to keep your heart rate flying!

- 16 × dumbbell fitball squats + dumbbell rows (16 right arm, 16 left arm) → **3 TIMES**
- 16 × alternating backward dumbbell lunge + fitball dumbbell chest press → **3 TIMES**
- 16 × step-ups with dumbbells (16 right leg, 16 left leg) + one-arm squat press → **3 TIMES**

HERO MOMENT 5-min run on treadmill, increase speed each minute!

ABS Do 16 reps of each exercise, the whole set 3 times through.
- lower body twist
- single leg extension
- plank on elbow (30 sec–1 min)

Day 3: wednesday: **fitness/cardio** *weigh-in day*

CLASS Body Attack, Spin, Boxing, Cardio Circuit, Dance **or CIRCUIT** ↓

RUN 45 mins. If you're struggling, aim for a slow jog rather than stopping to walk. If you *have* to walk, give yourself no more than 2 mins and get back to running. A good place to start is to run for 1 min and walk for 1½ mins. Record your distance and time on your Fitness Results Page. At a base level of fitness you should be covering 4–5km in 1 hour; upper levels closer to 7km.

ABS Do 16 reps of each exercise, the whole set 3 times through.
- bicycle
- side plank (right elbow), thread the needle
- side plank (left elbow), thread the needle

Day 4: thursday: **toning/strength**

CLASS Body Pump, strength/weights-based class **or**
SUPER SETS ↓ Do 16 reps of each exercise and perform each super set 3 times through before moving on to the next.

- 16 × squat with barbell + body rows → **3 TIMES**
- 16 × walking lunge with dumbbells (8 down, 8 back) + push-ups (knees or toes) → **3 TIMES**
- 16 × dynamic backward lunge on low step (16 right leg, 16 left leg) + one-arm squat press (16 right arm, 16 left arm) → **3 TIMES**

HERO MOMENT 500m rowing machine sprint

ABS Do 16 reps of each exercise, the whole set 3 times through.
- turkish get-ups (right-hand dumbbell)
- fitball crunches
- turkish get-ups (left-hand dumbbell)

FULL BODY STRETCH

Day 5: friday: **core & stretch**

WARM-UP
10-min jog

CLASS Yoga, Pilates **or**
CIRCUIT ↓ Perform 16 reps of each exercise, the whole set 3 times through.

- fitball back extension with shoulder blade squeeze
- fitball alternating back extension
- fitball aeroplane
- hand plank with twist
- plank on elbow (1-min)
- double crunch

FULL BODY STRETCH hold each stretch for at least 1 min and repeat sequence

Day 6: super saturday: **fitness/cardio**

WARM-UP
2-min jog, plus stretch hamstrings and calves

CLASS Mix two like Body Attack and Body Pump **or CIRCUIT** ↓

RUN You have a day off tomorrow, so come out guns blazing and give it your all! Your minimum training time is 1 hour, so aim for 1½ hours. This could be a mix of running and walking for 60 mins, followed by one round of Monday's circuit, abs and stretch, *or* simply run/walk for 1½ hours (e.g. 1-min run, 1-min walk). You *must* record your distance and time. At a base level you should aim to cover 5–6km in 1 hour; upper levels 7–8km.

FULL BODY STRETCH

Day 7: sunday: **rest**

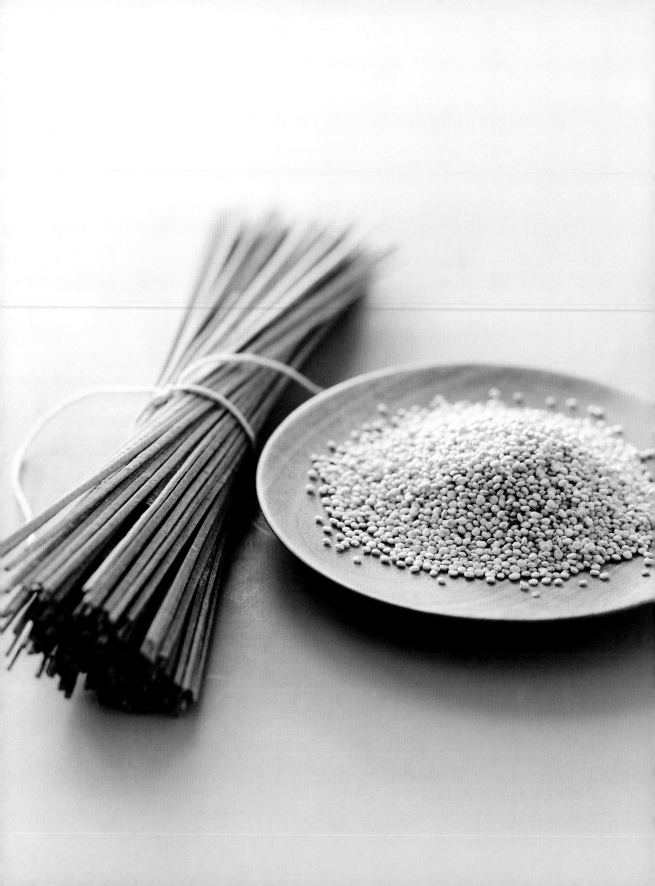

week 2

Take on what you have learnt about your behaviours this week and be brave and smart enough to learn from them. You are breaking old, poor habits and replacing them with new smart habits; however, it takes consistency and repetition. Long term efforts equal big results. Head into week 2 with a strengthened resolve!

My recommitment throughout this week is _____

shopping list and menu plan

Asparagus

Avocados

Beans, green

Beef fillets

Berries, fresh, mixed

Bok Choy, baby

Bream, whole

Broccolini

Capsicums, green

Capsicums, red

Carrots

Cauliflower

Celeriac

Chicken, breast fillets

Chillies, long red

Choy sum

Coriander

Corn on the cob

Cottage cheese

Cucumbers, Lebanese

Dill

Eggplant

Fennel

Flathead fillets

Garlic chives

Kangaroo, fillets

Lemons

Limes

Mint

Mushrooms, shiitake

Parsley

Prawns, raw, medium

Pumpkin

Ricotta, low-fat/lo-cal

Rocket

Shallots

Smoked salmon

Snapper, fillets

Spinach, baby

Spinach, English

Strawberries

Tempeh

Tomatoes

Tomatoes, roma

Tomatoes, sundried

Witlof

Wombok

Yoghurt, plain,
low-fat/lo-cal

Yoghurt, vanilla,
low-fat/lo-cal

Zucchinis

Remember, men can add a little more protein to each meal to make a total of 1800 calories per day, including snacks. Women: 1200 calories per day!

	breakfast	lunch	dinner	total cals
monday STIRFRY NIGHT	Special K, fruit, yoghurt and low-fat milk 259 cal	Spiced chargrilled vegetables with minted cracked wheat (leftovers from Sunday lunch) 281 cal	Stir-fried choy sum with chicken and soba noodles (make extra chicken for lunch tomorrow, no extra noodles) 293 cal	**833** **+ 367** *cal for snacks*
tuesday ACCELERATOR DAY! Snacks are vegies only today	Four egg-white omelette 300 cal	Cucumber, beetroot chicken and mint salad (using the leftover chicken from Sunday night dinner) 259 cal	Kangaroo with grilled capsicum, cucumber, baby rocket and witlof salad 300 cal	**859** **+ 341** *cal for snacks (vegies only)*
wednesday WEIGH-IN DAY!	Special K, fruit, yoghurt and low-fat milk 259 cals	Leftover curry from last week **or** Cauliflower and celeriac Madras curry 269 cal	Poached chicken, broad bean, chickpea and sundried tomato salad 302 cal	**830** **+ 370** *cal for snacks*
thursday	Quinoa porridge with cranberries and raisins 331 cal	Smoked salmon and salad wrap 302 cal	Chermoula prawn kebabs with couscous 301 cal	**934** **+ 266** *cal for snacks*
friday CURRY NIGHT	Special K, fruit, yoghurt and low-fat milk 259 cal	Tuna wrap **or** Stir-fried snapper with asparagus, wombok and shiitake mushrooms 260 cal	Cumin and chilli roasted vegetables with roasted garlic yoghurt (make up plenty of this and freeze in portions for next week's dinners or lunches) 269 cal	**788** **+ 412** *cal for snacks*
saturday	Scrambled egg whites with tempeh, shallots and diced tomato 344 cal	Dukkah-crusted flathead fillets with braised fennel and lemon 274 cal	Beef fillet with coriander salsa 302 cal	**920** **+ 280** *cal for snacks*
sunday	Fluffy buckwheat pancakes with berries and yoghurt 329 cal	Oven-baked whole bream with garlic spinach 299 cal **and** Watercress, fetta and watermelon salad 244 cal	Pan-fried chicken with steamed asian greens 303 cal	**1175** *no snacks needed today*

workout program

Day 8: monday: **fitness/cardio**

CLASS Body Attack, Spin, Boxing, Cardio Circuit, Dance **or**
CIRCUIT ↓ Perform 3 times through, with a 1½-min rest between each round.

<table>
<tr><td>WARM-UP
5-min jog</td><td><ul><li>2 laps of 400m oval or 800m on a treadmill or 4-min park run</li><li>16 × jumping jacks</li><li>16 × triceps dips off a bench</li><li>16 × mountain climbers</li><li>16 × fast low-step running right leg</li><li>16 × push-ups (knees or toes)</li><li>16 × fast low-step running left leg</li></ul>HERO MOMENT sprint around 400m oval or run the full length around your park. Time yourself.</td><td>ABS Do 16 reps of each exercise, the whole set 3 times through.<ul><li>crunches</li><li>twisting crunch to right</li><li>twisting crunch to left</li></ul></td><td>FULL BODY STRETCH</td></tr>
</table>

Day 9: tuesday: **toning/strength** *accelerator day*

CLASS Body Pump, strength/weights-based class **or**
SUPER SETS ↓ Do 16 reps of each exercise and each super set 3 times.
The jumping exercises at the end of each super set will give you a heart rate spike.

<table>
<tr><td>WARM-UP
5-min jog</td><td><ul><li>16 × dumbbell fitball squats + dumbbell rows (16 right arm, 16 left arm) + 10 × ice skaters → 3 TIMES</li><li>16 × alternating backward dumbbell lunges + fitball dumbbell chest press + 10 × plyometric lunges → 3 TIMES</li><li>16 × step-ups with dumbbells (16 right leg, 16 left leg) + one-arm squat press + 10 × frog jumps → 3 TIMES</li></ul>HERO MOMENT 5-min run on treadmill, increase speed each minute!</td><td>ABS Do 16 reps of each exercise, the whole set 3 times through.<ul><li>lower body twist</li><li>single leg extension</li><li>plank on elbow (30 sec–1 min)</li></ul></td><td>FULL BODY STRETCH</td></tr>
</table>

Day 10: wednesday: **fitness/cardio** *weigh-in day*

CLASS Body Attack, Spin, Boxing, Cardio Circuit, Dance **or CIRCUIT** ↓

<table>
<tr><td>WARM-UP
2-min jog, plus stretch hamstrings and calves</td><td>RUN 45 mins. Aim to improve your distance and/or your time compared to last Wednesday. Get out there and rip it up! Also, record your time and distance. At base level you should be reaching 5–6km; upper levels closer to 8km.</td><td>ABS Do 16 reps of each exercise, the whole set 3 times through.<ul><li>bicycle</li><li>side plank (right elbow) thread the needle</li><li>side plank (left elbow) thread the needle</li></ul></td><td>FULL BODY STRETCH</td></tr>
</table>

Day 11: thursday: **toning/strength**

WARM-UP
5-min jog

CLASS Body Pump, strength/weights-based class **or**
SUPER SETS ↓ Do 16 reps of each exercise and each super set 3 times.
The jumping exercises at the end of each super set will give you a heart rate spike.

- 16 × squats with barbell + body rows + 10 × ski jumps → **3 TIMES**
- 16 × walking lunge with dumbbells (8 down, 8 back) +
  push-ups (knees or toes) + 10 × ice skaters → **3 TIMES**
- 16 × dynamic backward lunges on low step (16 right leg,
  16 left leg) + one-arm squat press (16 right arm, 16 left arm) +
  10 × jumping jacks → **3 TIMES**

HERO MOMENT 500m rowing machine sprint

ABS Do 16 reps of each exercise, the whole set 3 times through.
- turkish get-ups (right-hand dumbbell)
- fitball crunches
- turkish get-ups (left-hand dumbbell)

FULL BODY STRETCH

Day 12: friday: **core & stretch**

WARM-UP
10-min jog

CLASS Yoga, Pilates **or**
CIRCUIT ↓ Perform 16 reps of each exercise, the whole set 3 times through.

- fitball back extension with shoulder blade squeeze
- fitball alternating back extension
- fitball aeroplane
- hand plank with twist
- plank on elbow (1-min)
- double crunch

FULL BODY STRETCH hold each stretch for at least 1-min and repeat sequence

Day 13: super saturday: **fitness/cardio**

WARM-UP
2-min jog, plus stretch hamstrings and calves

CLASS Mix two like Body Attack and Body Pump **or CIRCUIT ↓**

FITNESS TEST Do it the same way as your original test (see page 56), using the same oval etc and record your results. The idea is to beat your scores, which should be *easy*!

RUN Now do *at least* 1 hour of cardio training: either a 1-hour run or a shorter run, plus one round of Monday's circuit. Don't forget to record your time and distance. At a base level you should be aiming for 5–7km in 1 hour; upper levels 7–9km.

FULL BODY STRETCH

Day 14: sunday: **rest**

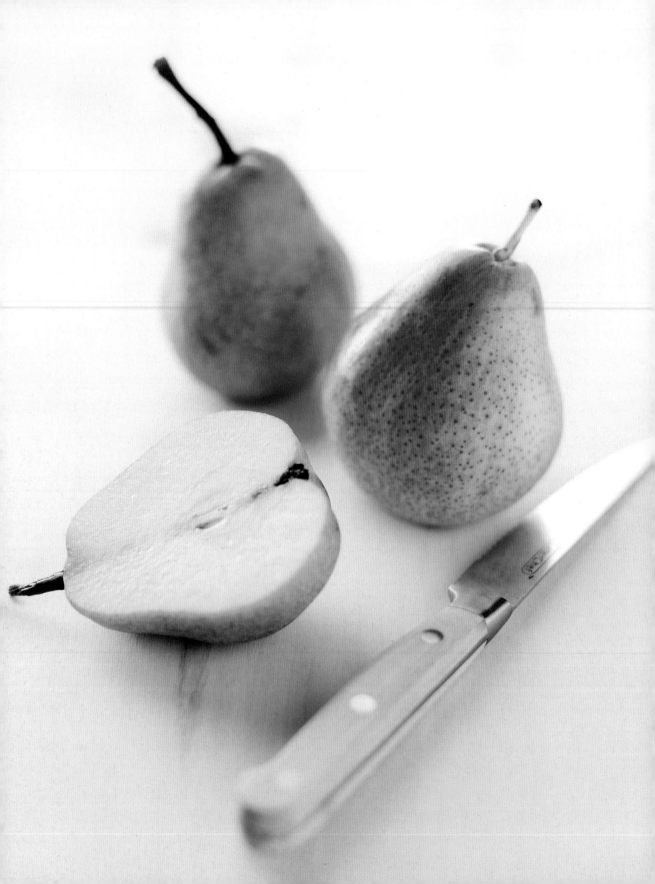

week 3

HALFWAY MARK! Be empowered by the choices you are making for yourself. Know that they will have repercussions for those around you, and of course for you! Every time you step up you are taking back control, living life and making things happen! At this point you should be seeing changes and facing new challenges.

My recommitment to week 3 is _____

shopping list and menu plan

Asparagus	Endive, curly	Snowpeas
Avocados	Fennel	Spinach, baby
Bananas	Fetta, low-fat/lo-cal	Spinach, English
Basil, fresh	Garlic chives	Strawberries
Berries, fresh, mixed	Grapefruit, pink, large	Tomatoes
Blueberries	Kangaroo fillets	Tomatoes, cherry
Bream, whole	Lemons	Tomatoes, roma
Broccolini	Limes	Tuna fillets
Capsicums, red	Mesclun	Witlof
Capsicums, yellow	Mint	Wombok
Carrots, baby	Mushrooms, field	Yoghurt, plain,
Carrots	Mushrooms, shiitake	low-fat/lo-cal
Cauliflower	Oregano	Yoghurt, vanilla,
Celeriac	Parsley	low-fat/lo-cal
Celery	Pears	Zucchinis
Chicken breast fillets	Prawns, raw, medium	
Chillies, long red	Pumpkin	
Chives	Radishes, red	
Choy sum	Ricotta, low-fat/lo-cal	
Coriander	Rocket	
Corn, baby	Scallops	
Cottage cheese	Shallots	
Cucumbers, Lebanese	Smoked salmon	
Dill	Snapper fillets	

Remember, men can add a little more protein to each meal to make a total of 1800 calories per day, including snacks. Women: 1200 calories per day!

	breakfast	lunch	dinner	total cals
monday STIRFRY NIGHT	Quinoa porridge with cranberries and raisins 331 cal	Chicken and salad wrap (use the extra chicken from last night's dinner) 302 cal	Stir-fried snapper with asparagus, wombok and shiitake mushrooms 260 cal	**893** **+ 307** *cal for snacks*
tuesday ACCELERATOR DAY!	Four egg-white omelette 300 cal	Pepper-crusted tuna with curly endive and cherry tomatoes 291 cal	Kangaroo with grilled capsicum, cucumber, baby rocket and witlof salad 300 cal	**891** **+ 309** *cal for snacks (vegies only)*
wednesday WEIGH-IN DAY!	Muesli, fruit and low-fat yoghurt 334 cal	Scallop, fennel and grapefruit salad 255 cal	Oven-baked whole bream with garlic spinach 299 cal	**888** **+ 312** *cal for snacks*
thursday	Boiled egg and soldiers 295 cal	Pear and walnut salad (add a small tin of tuna in spring water to this salad if you are extra hungry) 248 cal + 100 cal	Stir-fried choy sum with chicken and soba noodles (cook some extra chicken for tomorrow's lunch) 293 cal	**936** **+ 264** *cal for snacks*
friday CURRY NIGHT	Quinoa porridge with cranberries and raisins 331 cal	Crunchy mixed vegetable salad with almond vinaigrette (add about 120 grams of chicken from last night's dinner to beef up this salad) 261 cal + 180 cal	Cauliflower and celeriac Madras curry 269 cal	**1041** **+ 159** *cal for snacks*
saturday	Fluffy buckwheat pancakes with berries and yoghurt 329 cal	Lentil salad with yellow capsicum, coriander and cranberries 302 cal	Steamed minted chicken with broccolini and baby carrots 279 cal	**910** **+ 290** *cal for snacks*
sunday	Pan-fried field mushrooms and tomatoes with fetta and oregano 310 cal	Chermoula prawn kebabs with couscous 301 cal	Cumin and chilli roasted vegetables with roasted garlic yoghurt (make up extra portions of these for lunch) 287 cal	**898** **+ 302** *cal for snacks*

workout program

Day 15: monday: **fitness/cardio**

CLASS Body Attack, Spin, Boxing, Cardio Circuit, Dance **or**
CIRCUIT ↓ Perform 3 times through with a 1½-min rest between each round.

- two laps of 400m oval *or* 800m on a treadmill *or* 4-min park run
- 16 × jumping jacks
- 16 × triceps dips off a bench
- 16 × mountain climbers
- 16 × frog jumps
- 16 × push-ups (knees or toes)
- 16 × ice skaters

HERO MOMENT one sprint around 400m oval *or* run the full length around your park. Time yourself.

ABS Do 16 reps of each exercise, the whole set 3 times through.
- crunches
- twisting crunch to right
- twisting crunch to left

Day 16: tuesday: **toning/strength** *accelerator day*

CLASS Body Pump, strength/weights-based class **or**
SUPER SETS ↓ Do 16 reps of each exercise and each super set 3 times.
The jumping exercises at the end of each super set will give you a heart rate spike.

- 16 × dumbbell fitball squats + dumbbell rows (16 right arm, 16 left arm) + 20 × over the fence jumps →**3 TIMES**
- 16 × alternating backward dumbbell lunges + fitball dumbbell chest press + 20 × plyometric lunges →**3 TIMES**
- 16 × step-ups with dumbbells (16 right leg, 16 left leg) + one-arm squat press + 20 × frog jumps →**3 TIMES**

HERO MOMENT 5-min run on treadmill, increase speed each minute!

ABS Do 16 reps of each exercise, the whole set 3 times through.
- lower body twist
- single leg extension
- plank on elbow (30 sec–1 min)

Day 17: wednesday: **fitness/cardio** *weigh-in day*

CLASS Body Attack, Spin, Boxing, Cardio Circuit, Dance **or CIRCUIT ↓**

RUN 45 mins. At this point you should be noticing a real difference due to being lighter and of course *fitter*! Please record your time and distance. At base level you should be reaching 5–7km; upper levels 8–9km.

ABS Do 16 reps of each exercise, the whole set 3 times through.
- bicycle
- side plank (right), thread the needle
- side plank (left), thread the needle

Day 18: thursday: **toning/strength**

WARM-UP
5-min jog

CLASS Body Pump, strength/weights-based class **or**
SUPER SETS ↓ Do 16 reps of each exercise and each super set 3 times.
The jumping exercises at the end of each super set will give you a heart rate spike.

- 16 × squats with barbell + body rows + 20 × ski jumps →**3 TIMES**
- 16 × walking lunges (8 down, 8 back) + push-ups (knees or toes) + 20 × ice skaters →**3 TIMES**
- 16 × dynamic backward lunge on low step (16 right leg, 16 left leg) + one-arm squat press (16 right arm, 16 left arm) + 20 × jumping jacks →**3 TIMES**

HERO MOMENT 500m rowing machine sprint

ABS Do 16 reps of each exercise, the whole set 3 times through.
- turkish get-ups (right-hand dumbbell)
- fitball crunches
- turkish get-ups (left-hand dumbbell)

FULL BODY STRETCH

Day 19: friday: **core & stretch**

WARM-UP
10-min jog

CLASS Yoga, Pilates **or**
CIRCUIT ↓ Perform 16 reps of each exercise, 3 times through.

- fitball back extension with shoulder blade squeeze
- fitball alternating back extension
- fitball aeroplanes
- hand plank with twist
- plank on elbow (1 min)
- double crunch

FULL BODY STRETCH hold each stretch for at least 1 min and repeat sequence

Day 20: super saturday: **fitness/cardio**

WARM-UP
2-min jog, plus stretch hamstrings and calves

CLASS Mix two like Body Attack and Body Pump **or CIRCUIT** ↓

RUN You've put in a lot of time and effort so this session will show you just how fit you've become. Your MINIMUM training time is 1½ hrs, so either run/jog for the whole time or run for 45 mins and follow it up with Monday's circuit. Please record your time and distance. At a base level you should be aiming for 6–8km in a 1-hour run; upper levels 8–10km. Obviously you'll cover more distance in 1½ hours.

FULL BODY STRETCH

Day 21: sunday: **rest**

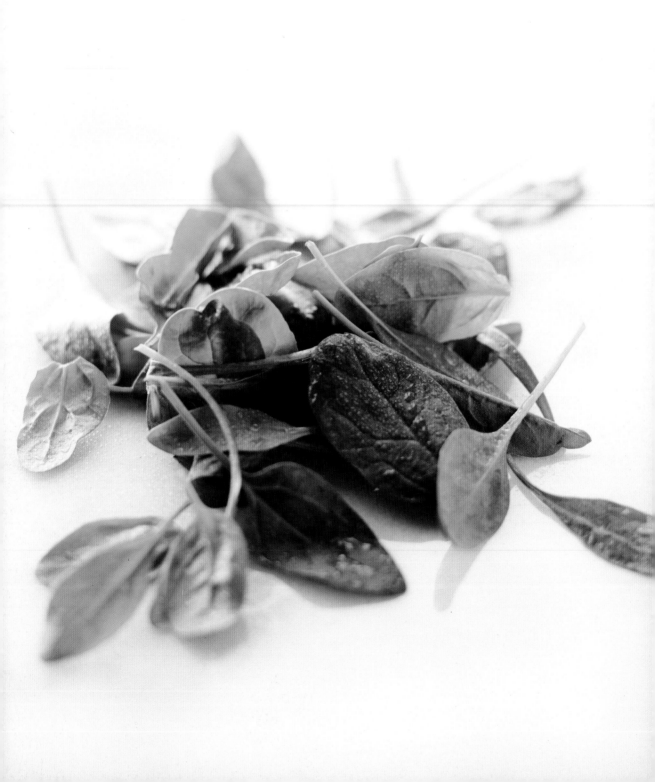

week 4

This is your week to lay down the gauntlet, search within and prove that you and your life are worth the effort. Find success in the valuable lessons you have learnt along the way. Be brave and be open to the challenges ahead in this last week.

My commitment to the end of this program and

for my future is _____

shopping list and menu plan

Avocados

Bananas

Beans, green

Beef, fillets

Berries, fresh, mixed

Blueberries

Bok Choy, baby

Bream, whole

Broccolini

Capsicums, green

Capsicums, red

Carrots

Chicken breast fillets

Chillies, long red

Choy sum

Coriander

Corn on the cob

Cottage cheese

Cucumbers, Lebanese

Dill

Eggplant

Fennel

Flathead fillets

Garlic chives

Grapefruit, pink

Kangaroo fillets

Lemons

Limes

Mint

Octopus, baby

Parsley

Pears

Pumpkin

Radishes, red

Ricotta, low-fat/lo-cal

Rocket

Scallops

Shallots

Smoked salmon

Spinach, baby

Spinach, English

Strawberries

Tempeh

Tomatoes

Tomatoes, baby roma

Tomatoes, roma

Witlof

Wombok

Yoghurt, plain,
   low-fat/lo-cal

Yoghurt, vanilla,
   low-fat/lo-cal

Zucchinis

Remember, men can add a little more protein to each meal to make a total of 1800 calories per day, including snacks. Women: 1200 calories per day!

	breakfast	lunch	dinner	total cals
monday STIRFRY NIGHT	Special K, fruit, yoghurt and low-fat milk 259 cal	Cumin and chilli roasted vegetables with roasted garlic yoghurt (leftovers from last night's dinner) 287 cal	Stir-fried choy sum with chicken and soba noodles 293 cal	**839** **+ 361** *cal for snacks*
tuesday ACCELERATOR DAY!	Four egg-white omelette 300 cal	Cucumber, beetroot, chicken and mint salad 259 cal	Kangaroo with grilled capsicum, cucumber, baby rocket and witlof salad 300 cal	**859** **+ 341** *cal for snacks (vegies only)*
wednesday WEIGH-IN DAY!	Muesli, fruit and low-fat yoghurt 334 cal	Smoked salmon and salad wrap 302 cal	Spiced chargrilled vegetables with minted cracked wheat (cook up extra portions for lunches) 281 cal	**917** **+ 283** *cal for snacks*
thursday	Special K, fruit, yoghurt and low-fat milk 259 cal	Thai octopus salad 247 cal	Oven-baked whole bream with garlic spinach 299 cal	**805** **+ 395** *cal for snacks*
friday CURRY NIGHT	Quinoa porridge with cranberries and raisins 331 cal	Spiced chargrilled vegetables with minted cracked wheat (leftovers from Wednesday night's dinner) 281 cal	Cumin and chilli roasted vegetables with roasted garlic yoghurt 287 cal	**899** **+ 301** *cal for snacks*
saturday	Scrambled egg whites with tempeh, shallots and diced tomato 344 cal	Dukkah-crusted flathead fillets with braised fennel and lemon 274 cal	Beef fillet with coriander salsa (cook up some extra beef for lunch on Monday) 302 cal	**920** **+ 280** *cal for snacks*
sunday	Fluffy buckwheat pancakes with berries and yoghurt 329 cal	Scallop, fennel and grapefruit salad 255 cal	Pan-fried chicken with steamed Asian greens 303 cal	**893** **+ 307** *cal for snacks*

workout program

Day 22: monday: **fitness/cardio**

CLASS Body Attack, Spin, Boxing, Cardio Circuit, Dance **or**
CIRCUIT ↓ Perform 3 times through with 1½-min rest between each round *or*
see if you can do it 4 TIMES!

<table>
<tr><td rowspan="2">WARM-UP
5-min jog</td><td>

- Two laps of 400m oval *or* 800m treadmill *or* 4-min park run
- 16 × jumping jacks
- 16 × triceps dips off a bench
- 16 × mountain climbers
- 16 × frog jumps
- 16 × push-ups (knees or toes)
- 16 × ice-skaters

HERO MOMENT one sprint around a 400m oval *or* run the full length around your park. Time yourself.

</td><td>

ABS Do 16 reps of each exercise, the whole set 3 times through.
- crunches
- twisting crunch to right
- twisting crunch to left

</td><td rowspan="2">FULL BODY STRETCH</td></tr>
</table>

Day 23: tuesday: **toning/strength** *accelerator day*

CLASS Body Pump, strength/weights-based class **or**
SUPER SETS ↓ Do 16 reps of each exercise and each super set 3 times.
The jumping exercises at the end of each super set will give you a heart rate spike.

<table>
<tr><td rowspan="2">WARM-UP
5-min jog</td><td>

- 16 × dumbbell fitball squats + dumbbell rows (16 right arm, 16 left arm) + 20 × over the fence jumps → **3 TIMES**
- 16 × alternating backward dumbbell lunges + fitball dumbbell chest press + 20 × plyometric lunges → **3 TIMES**
- 16 × step-ups with dumbbells (16 right leg, 16 left) + standing dumbbell shoulder press + 20 × frog jumps → **3 TIMES**

HERO MOMENT 5-min run on treadmill, increase speed *and incline* each minute!

</td><td>

ABS Do 16 reps of each exercise, the whole set 3 times through.
- lower body twist
- single leg extension
- plank on elbow (30 sec–1 min)

</td><td rowspan="2">FULL BODY STRETCH</td></tr>
</table>

Day 24: wednesday: **fitness/cardio** *weigh-in day + body measurement*

CLASS Body Attack, Spin, Boxing, Cardio Circuit, Dance **or CIRCUIT** ↓

<table>
<tr><td rowspan="2">WARM-UP
2-min jog, plus stretch hamstrings and calves</td><td>

RUN 45 mins. Today's main aim is to improve your distance or your time or both in comparison to last Wednesday. This is your last run before the BIG ONE, so go for it! At base level you should be reaching 5–7km; at upper levels 8–9km.

</td><td>

ABS Do 16 reps of each exercise, and the whole set 3 times through.
- bicycle
- side plank (right), thread the needle
- side plank (left), thread the needle

</td><td rowspan="2">FULL BODY STRETCH</td></tr>
</table>

Day 25: thursday: **toning/strength**

WARM-UP
5-min jog

CLASS Body Pump, strength/weights-based class **or**
SUPER SETS ↓ Do 16 reps of each exercise and each super set 3 times. The jumping exercises at the end of each super set will give you a heart rate spike. Go HARD here! You know these exercises now and you know how to get the best out of yourself, so make it happen!

- 16 × squats with barbell + body rows + 20 × ski jumps → **3 TIMES**
- 16 × walking lunges (8 down, 8 back) + push-ups (knees or toes) + 20 × ice skaters → **3 TIMES**
- 16 × dynamic backward lunge on low step (16 right leg, 16 left leg) + one-arm squat press (16 right arm, 16 left arm) + 20 × jumping jacks → **3 TIMES**

HERO MOMENT 500m rowing machine sprint

ABS Do 16 reps of each exercise, the whole set 3 times through.
- turkish get-ups (right-hand dumbbell)
- fitball crunches
- turkish get-ups (left-hand dumbbell)

FULL BODY STRETCH

Day 26: friday: **core & stretch**

WARM-UP
10-min jog

CLASS Yoga, Pilates **or**
CIRCUIT ↓ Perform 16 reps of each exercise, 3 times through.

- fitball back extension with shoulder blade squeeze
- fitball alternating back extension
- fitball aeroplane
- hand plank with twist
- plank on elbow (1-min)
- double crunch

FULL BODY STRETCH hold each stretch for at least 1 min and repeat sequence

Day 27: super saturday: **fitness/cardio**

WARM-UP
2-min jog, plus stretch hamstrings and calves

CLASS Mix two like Body Attack and Body Pump **or CIRCUIT** ↓

RUN This is our *last* Super Saturday session, so of course I'm upping the stakes! Today everyone must do 10km, and focus on running more than walking. Remember, if you feel like walking, slow your pace to a shuffle and focus on breathing. You can *always* do more than you think, so think big! If you've already been clocking close to 10km on other Super Saturdays, you should be aiming for 15km. Good luck!

FULL BODY STRETCH

Day 28: sunday: **rest**

Day 29: monday: **fitness/cardio**

WARM-UP 5-min jog

CLASS Body Attack, Spin, Boxing, Cardio Circuit, Dance **or**
CIRCUIT ↓ Perform 3 times through with 1½-min rest between each round *or* see if you can do it FOUR TIMES!

- Two laps of 400m oval *or* 800m treadmill *or* 4-min park run
- 16 × jumping jacks
- 16 × triceps dips off a bench
- 16 × mountain climbers
- 16 × frog jumps
- 16 × push-ups (knees or toes)
- 16 × ice-skaters

HERO MOMENT one sprint around a 400m oval *or* run the full length around your park. Time yourself.

ABS Do 16 reps of each exercise, the whole set 3 times through.
- crunches
- twisting crunch to right
- twisting crunch to left

FULL BODY STRETCH

	breakfast	lunch	dinner	total cals
monday	Muesli, fruit and low-fat yoghurt 334 cal	Pear and walnut salad 248 cal	Stir-fried choy sum with chicken and soba noodles 293 cal	875 **+ 325** *cal for snacks*

Day 30: tuesday: **final fitness test & weigh-in + body measurements**

FITNESS TEST: Take this in exactly the same way you did at the start and on Day 13, and then complete the *biggest* cardio session of your life. Today is the very last day of this challenge, and your chance to prove to yourself just how amazing you have become over the last 30 days!

Maintenance plan

Wow, you look amazing! Now you have shown just what you are capable of! And that person has always been inside of you. I am excited for your future and your next fitness challenges. But be careful: one of the biggest traps I see when people reach their goal weight is that they assume they can go back to their old habits. Or little by little those sneaky treats start to happen, and training sessions get blown off. This is when you will see the return of the weight – it's that simple. **The fact that you've reached your goal weight does not change anything!** You will always be an exerciser, and you will always choose to eat well. This way, you'll always be at your goal weight. Personally, I tend to loosen the reins a little on the weekend, but I always maintain my training so I can stay pretty much the same weight all the time. But it's more than that: I can live a life full of energy and vitality. This is something that everyone can do – **it's up to you to choose it**. To stay at your goal weight there are a few simple things you need to do. This has been a really intense 30 days so to maintain an exercise program longer term, you should aim to train six days a week (which usually means you will manage five training sessions). You can also pull back on the intensity of each training session. I recommend maintaining the daily calorie counts during the week but you can go easier at the weekend. If you see the scales creeping back up, you know the rules: check in on portion sizes and calorie counts, pull back on alcohol and be consistent in your training.

snacks

When it comes to snacks people tend to get in trouble with portion sizes. A snack is just that, a snack! It's a small something; just to tide you over till your next meal. It can be any sort of wholefood as long as it is low in fat and comes in at round 100 to 150 calories. Always check in with yourself before snacking. Is the need for a snack about boredom and therefore simply a habit?

Here are my healthy snack suggestions:

- Bowl of strawberries (250 grams): 70 cal - 20 frozen grapes are great on a hot summer's day: 80 cal - 2 long sticks of celery dipped in 2 tablespoons of hummus: 100 cal - 1 ½ cups edamame (in pods, no salt): 100 cal - 1 cup freshly squeezed orange juice, frozen. It's just like a sorbet: 110 cal - 2 thickly sliced pear discs with a tablespoon low-fat ricotta cheese, mint and ground cinnamon and a cup of tea: 120 cal - Mixed berry frappe – throw 1 cup frozen mixed berries, 3 tablespoons low-fat yoghurt and 4 ice cubes into a blender: 140 cal - Homemade icypoles made from low-fat yoghurt and fruit: 80 cal - 2 large iceberg lettuce leaves with ½ cup shredded chicken (put aside from last night's chicken stirfry) and a tablespoon tomato salsa in each: 150 cal - 2 cups air-popped popcorn (no salt, no butter – try adding spices like ground cinnamon or chilli instead): 60 cal.

Quinoa porridge with cranberries and raisins

This porridge is delicious and very filling. The cranberries and raisins give it a lovely hit of sweetness, and the walnuts add richness. This would have to be one of my all-time favourite breakfasts.

Serves 2
Prep 5 minutes
Cook 20 minutes
331 cal per serve

¾ cup quinoa, rinsed and drained

500 ml water

375 ml low-cal milk

⅓ cup dried cranberries

2 tablespoons raisins

¼ cup coarsely chopped walnuts

1. Combine the quinoa and water in a saucepan and bring to the boil. Reduce the heat to medium–low and cook, covered, for 10 minutes.

2. Stir in 1 cup of the milk and the dried fruit and nuts. Cook, covered, for another 10 minutes, then stir in the remaining milk.

TIPS

- Quinoa originates from South America. The Incas held this crop sacred and referred to it as 'the mother of all grain'. It's actually a plant related to spinach and silverbeet. We're using the seeds here; the leaves are also edible but they're not available in Australia.

- Quinoa has a nutty flavour and a high protein content. It's gluten free, a good source of iron and magnesium, easy to prepare and yummy . . . what's not to like?

- Although most quinoa comes pre-rinsed, it's a good idea to rinse it under cold water until the water runs clear, and then drain it. This removes any outer coating, which has a bitter taste.

- Quinoa absorbs a lot of liquid, so the amount of milk you add depends on how you like your porridge. Check after 20 minutes and if the consistency is right, don't add the remaining ½ cup milk (308 calories per serve).

- For a tasty variation, try adding a grated apple and a sliced banana with the walnuts, instead of the dried fruit (313 calories per serve).

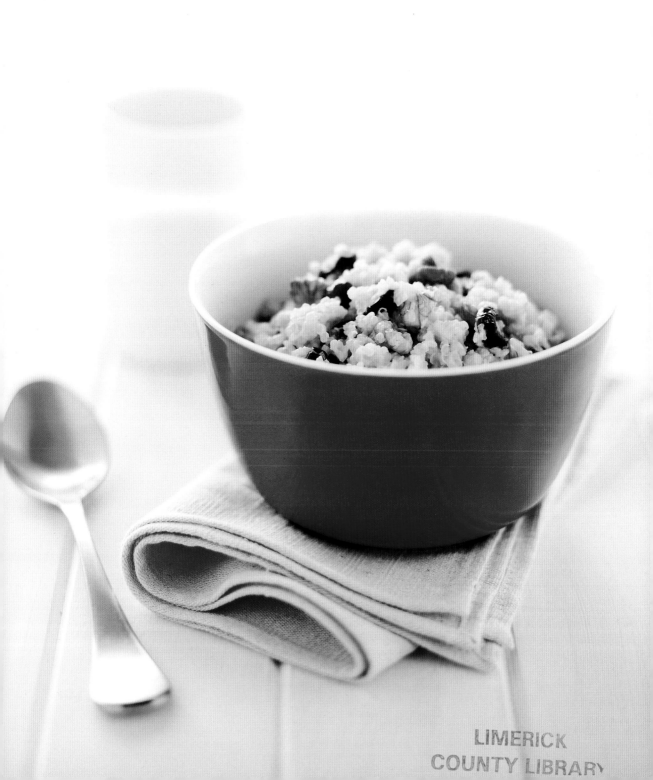

Four egg-white omelette

This is one of my essential recipes: quick to make and perfect for a solid protein burst.

Serves 1
Prep 5 minutes
Cook 3 minutes
300 cal per serve

light olive oil spray
4 egg whites
1 tablespoon cottage cheese
120 g smoked salmon or
    tuna in springwater
1 tablespoon chopped chives

1. Heat a frying pan and spray with light olive oil spray. Add the egg whites and roll the pan so the egg whites evenly cover the base of the pan. Cook on low heat for 3 minutes.

2. When the sides of the omelette lift easily, add a dollop of cottage cheese to the middle and fold the omelette over on itself. Top with the smoked salmon and chives.

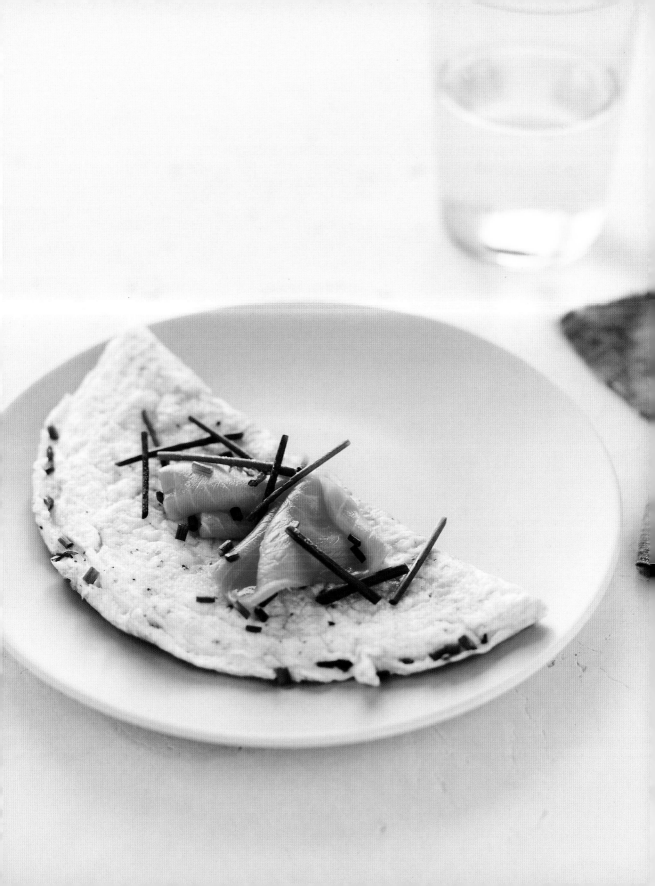

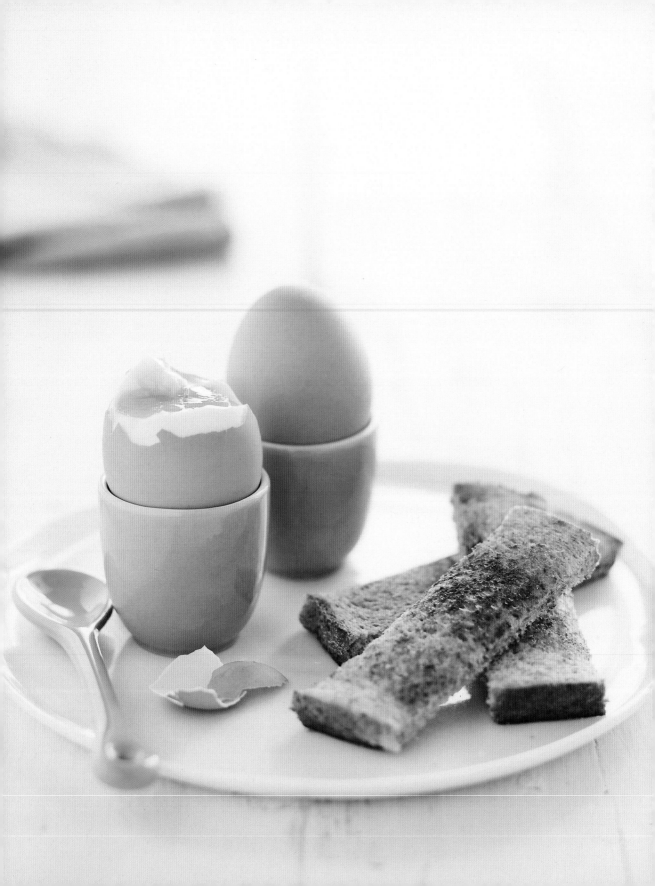

Boiled egg and soldiers

Old-fashioned comfort food to set you up for the day ahead.
(The picture shows a serve for two.)

1 egg
2 slices wholegrain toast

Serves 1
Prep 5 minutes
Cook 20 minutes
255 cal per serve

1. Bring a saucepan of water to the boil, then simmer the egg for 5 minutes. Slice the toast into 1 cm strips and dip in the egg. Spead the toast with 2 tablespoons low-fat cottage cheese for an extra protein burst (adds 40 cal).

Michelle's favourite fast breakfasts

These are my absolute staples for a weekday breakfast. A small amount of cereal, lots of fruit and a good dollop of yoghurt will fill you up.

Muesli
¼ cup untoasted muesli, with 1 banana, 6 strawberries, ⅓ punnet blueberries and
½ cup (100 g) low-fat yoghurt (334 cal)

Special K
¾ cup Special K, with 125 ml low-fat or soy milk, 6 strawberries and
¼ cup low-fat yoghurt (259 cal)

Scrambled egg whites with tempeh, shallots and diced tomato

I love the idea of a hot brekkie – it makes me feel as though I'm having something really special for breakfast. Tempeh is such a fabulous product; it has a nice 'chew' factor and a lovely smoky flavour. The shallots kick the flavour along and you can't beat tomatoes for great antioxidants. This is food to keep you young!

Serves 2
Prep 10 minutes
Cook 10 minutes
344 cal per serve

olive oil spray
180 g tempeh, cut into cubes
2 shallots, thinly sliced
1 clove garlic, crushed
1 tomato, diced
freshly cracked black pepper

6 egg whites, lightly beaten
¼ cup low-cal ricotta
2 tablespoons coarsely chopped parsley
2 slices wholegrain bread, toasted

1. Spray a non-stick frying pan with oil and heat on medium. Cook the tempeh for 2–3 minutes or until golden and heated through. Add the shallots and garlic and cook, stirring, until the shallots start to soften. Stir through the tomato and season with pepper.

2. Meanwhile, spray a small saucepan with oil. Cook the egg whites until they start to set. Remove from the heat and stir through the ricotta and half the parsley. Season with pepper.

3. Serve the scrambled egg whites with toast and the tempeh mixture. Sprinkle over the remaining parsley.

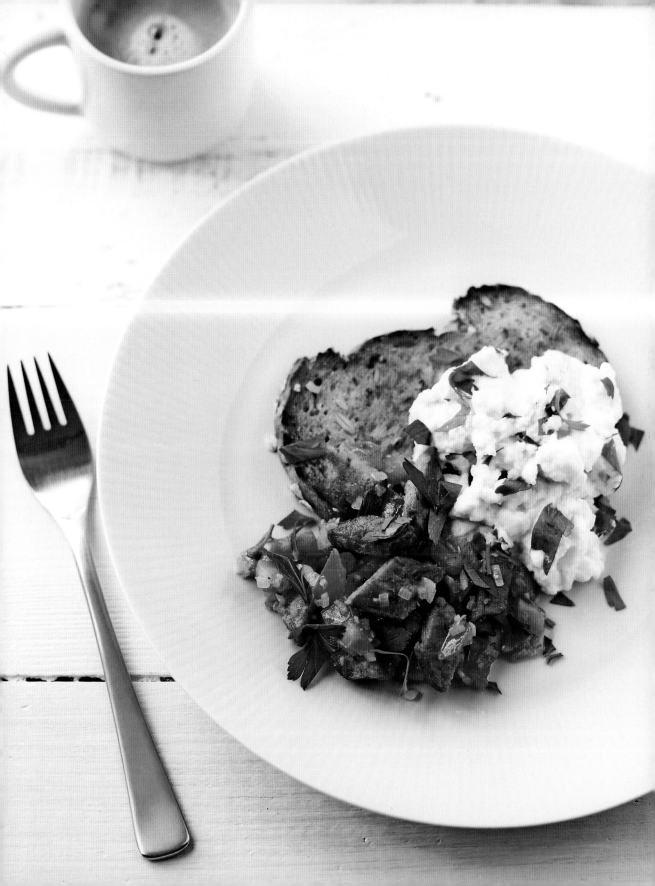

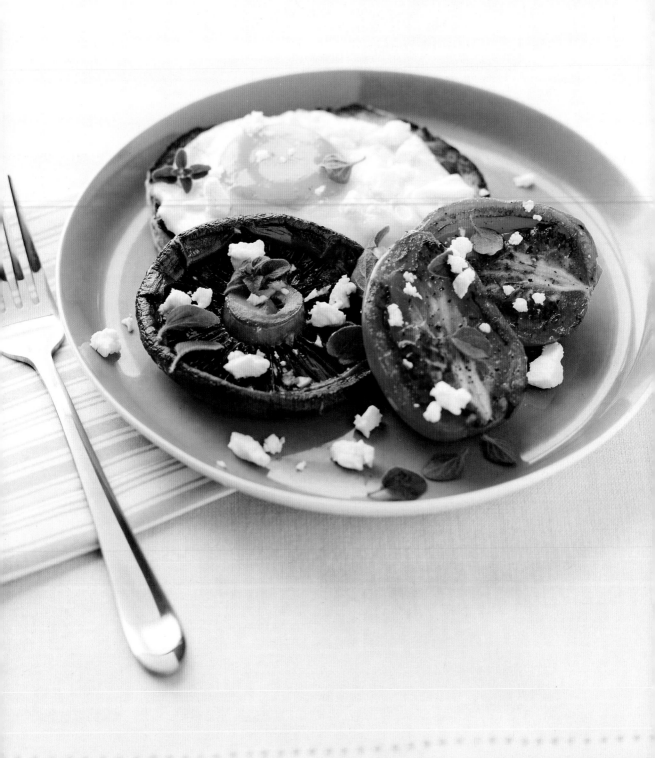

Pan-fried field mushrooms and tomatoes with fetta and oregano

Good field mushrooms can be as sustaining as eating a piece of steak – thick, chewy, juicy and hearty. Add some melt-in-the-mouth fetta and fresh oregano, and you could be tricked into thinking you are sitting at your local cafe.

olive oil spray

2 field mushrooms

2 roma tomatoes, halved

2 large eggs

1 clove garlic, crushed

50 g low-cal fetta

1 tablespoon small oregano leaves

freshly cracked black pepper

2 slices rye bread

Serves 2

Prep 5 minutes

Cook 15 minutes

310 cal per serve

1. Spray a large non-stick frying pan with oil and heat on medium. Cook the mushrooms, covered, for about 5 minutes. Increase the heat to medium–high, add the tomatoes and cook for 3–4 minutes.

2. Crack the eggs into the pan and cook for about 2 minutes until the vegetables are tender and the eggs are cooked. Add the garlic to the mushrooms and turn to coat.

3. Divide between two plates and sprinkle the vegetables with the fetta and oregano. Season with pepper and serve with the rye bread.

TIPS

- Big field mushrooms take time to cook. If you're in a hurry, you could use the same weight of small button mushrooms.

- If your pan isn't big enough to fit all the ingredients, cook the eggs separately in a small pan.

- If you're not into eggs, cook 2 mushrooms per person instead and increase the fetta to 80 g (294 calories per serve).

Fluffy buckwheat pancakes with berries and yoghurt

Um, pancakes? In a weight-loss book? Yep! These babies are fantastic, not just for you but for the whole family – get the kids involved and they are even more likely to eat them. Fresh berries are a must.

Serves 4
Prep 10 minutes
Cook 15 minutes
329 cal per serve

1 cup low-cal ricotta
1 egg
310 ml low-cal milk
½ cup buckwheat flour
½ cup self-raising wholemeal flour

cooking oil spray
400 g fresh mixed berries
1 cup low-cal vanilla yoghurt

1. Whisk the ricotta, egg and milk in a large bowl until smooth. Whisk in the flours.

2. Lightly spray a non-stick frying pan with oil and heat on medium. Pour a generous eighth of the pancake mixture into the pan. Cook for 2–3 minutes each side until golden and puffed. Transfer to a plate and keep warm while you cook the other pancakes. Wipe the pan with paper towel and cook the remaining batter.

3. Serve the warm pancakes immediately, with the berries and yoghurt.

TIPS

● This recipe makes 8 pancakes. If there are only two of you eating, reserve half of the ricotta, egg and milk mixture and store it, covered, in the refrigerator for the next day. Whisk ¼ cup each of buckwheat and self-raising wholemeal flour into the remaining ricotta mixture and proceed with the recipe. Serve with half the berries and yoghurt.

● Each pancake without topping is about 125 calories.

● You can store cooled cooked pancakes in an airtight container and reheat them in the microwave, but they will not have such a light and fluffy texture.

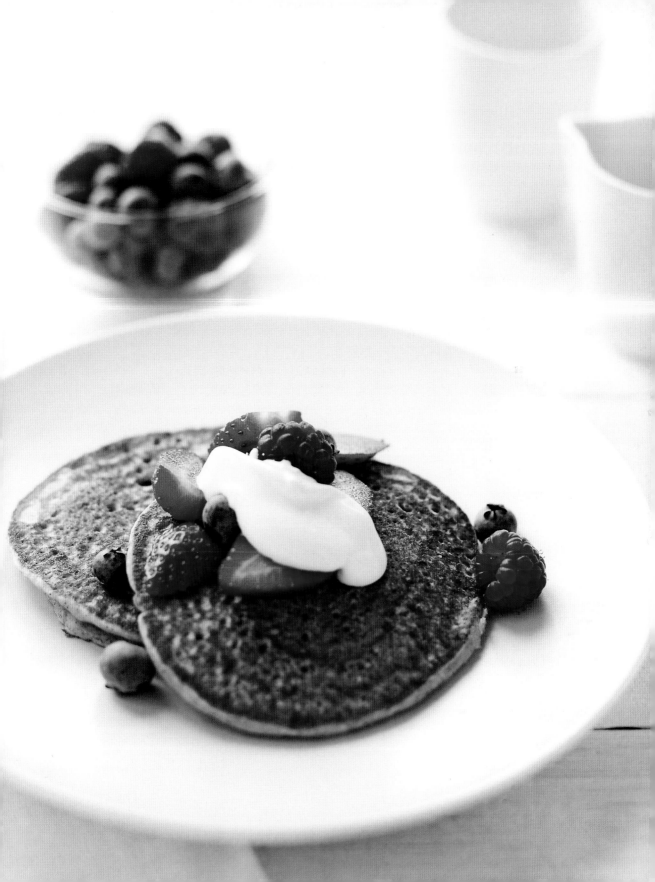

Smoked salmon and salad wrap

This is such a great basic recipe – have it every day for an easy lunch, and for variation swap the smoked salmon for tinned salmon or tuna (both in springwater) or leftover chicken. (This makes enough for 2, so halve the ingredients if you are just making it for yourself.)

Serves 2
Prep 10 minutes
302 cal per serve

2 wholemeal flatbreads/
   mountain breads
1 tablespoon wholegrain mustard
170 g smoked salmon
½ small avocado, mashed

1 carrot, coarsely grated
1 tomato, sliced
2 handfuls baby rocket or spinach
1 tablespoon chopped dill

1. Spread the bread with mustard, then pile high with salmon and salad. Sprinkle with dill. Roll up and serve.

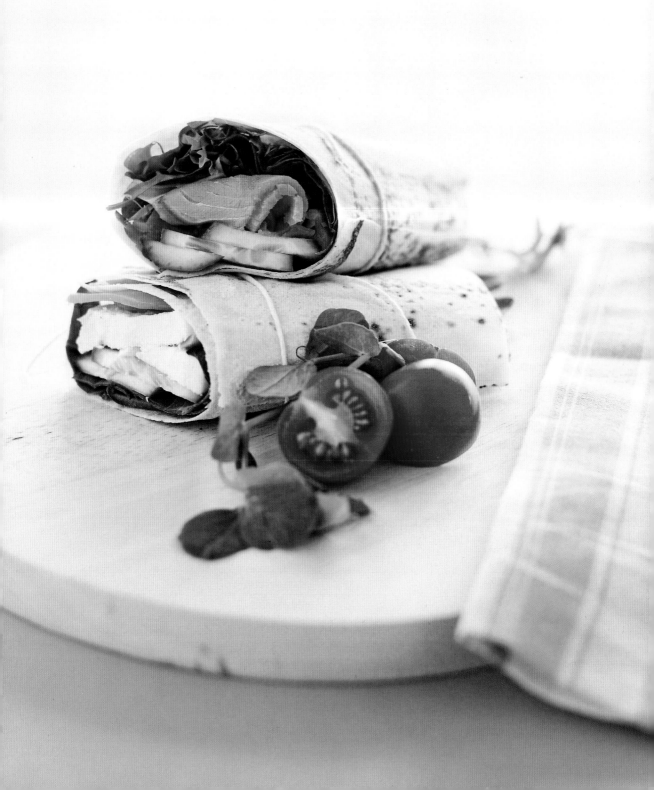

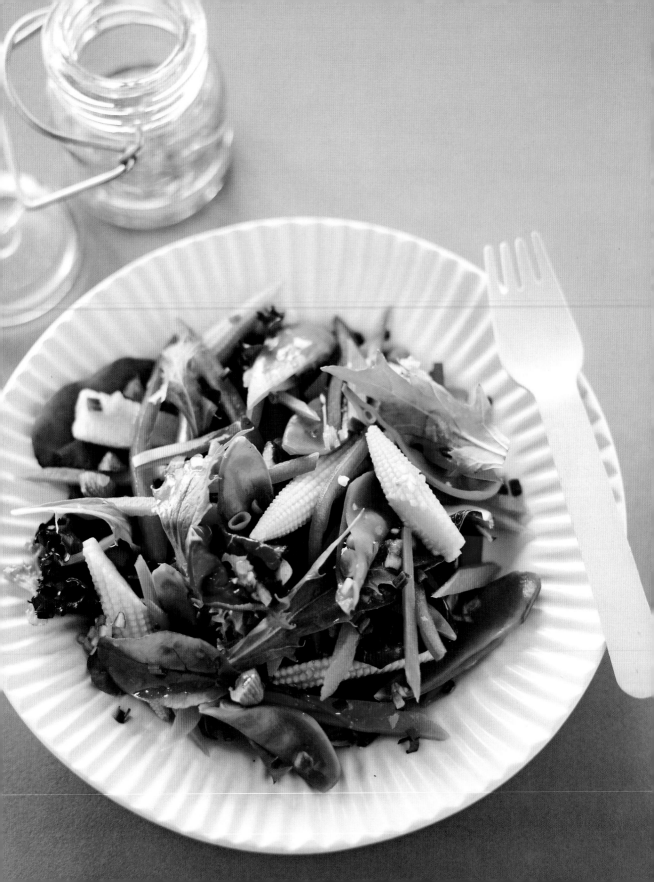

Crunchy mixed vegetable salad with almond vinaigrette

This fresh, simple salad with a tangy, crisp dressing is the perfect accompaniment to a dish. You can make it a main meal by adding sliced chicken or beef.

125 g baby corn
125 g snowpeas, trimmed
80 g mesclun
1 small carrot, julienned
1 red capsicum, thinly sliced
½ shallot, finely chopped

1 tablespoon red wine vinegar
2 teaspoons extra virgin olive oil
2 tablespoons finely chopped chives
freshly cracked black pepper
2 tablespoons coarsely chopped
    roasted almonds

Serves 2
Prep 10 minutes
261 cal per serve

1. Cook the corn in a small saucepan of boiling water for 2 minutes. Add the snowpeas and bring to the boil. Cook for 1 minute. Drain and cool in iced water. Drain again.

2. Halve or quarter the corn. Slice the snowpeas on the diagonal.

3. Combine the corn, snowpeas, mesclun, carrot and capsicum in a salad bowl.

4. Make a dressing by combining the shallot, vinegar, oil and half the chives in a small bowl. Season.

5. Drizzle the dressing over the salad and gently toss to coat. Sprinkle with the almonds and remaining chives.

TIPS

- Shallots are often called eschalots or French shallots, as they are very popular in France. They look like small onions. Their flesh is purple and they are sweeter and milder than onions, which makes them ideal for eating raw in salads.

- You can add 125 g cooked chicken breast (322 calories per serve) for a main meal.

Lentil salad with yellow capsicum, coriander and cranberries

Sometimes I don't feel like eating a meat dish at night, and this great vegetarian salad is perfect. The health properties of lentils are enormous and they definitely leave you feeling full. The cranberries add a lovely hint of sweetness.

Serves 2
Prep 10 minutes
Cook 35 minutes
302 cal per serve

⅔ cup French-style green lentils, rinsed and drained
1 large stick celery, thinly sliced
1 yellow capsicum, cut into cubes
100 g cherry tomatoes, halved
⅓ cup coarsely chopped coriander

1 tablespoon lemon juice
2 teaspoons extra virgin olive oil
1 clove garlic, crushed
freshly cracked black pepper
2 tablespoons dried cranberries

1. Cook the lentils in a small saucepan of gently boiling water for 30–35 minutes or until tender. Drain and rinse.

2. Combine the lentils with the celery, capsicum, tomatoes and coriander in a salad bowl.

3. Make a dressing by combining the lemon juice, oil and garlic in a small bowl. Season.

4. Drizzle the dressing over the salad and gently toss to coat. Sprinkle with the cranberries.

TIPS

- French-style green lentils are grown in Australia. The small dark-green lentils don't disintegrate when they're cooked, which makes them ideal for salads.

- As with all pulses, lentils need to be cooked in non-salted water, as salt prevents them from softening. If you're using canned lentils, you'll need about 1½ cups.

- If you're not keen on cranberries, leave them out (260 calories per serve).

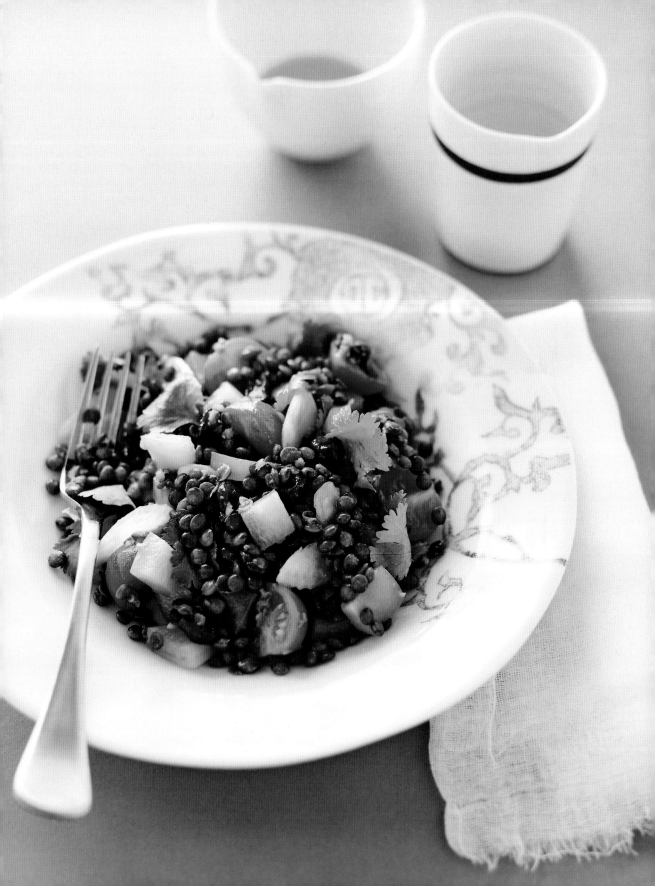

Pear and walnut salad

The combination of pear and walnut makes a fresh, clean, tasty salad. It takes very little time to prepare, which makes it a popular choice to make in the morning and take to work. It's also super low in calories but super high in taste.

Serves 2

Prep 10 minutes

248 cal per serve

2 pears, unpeeled, cored and
  thinly sliced

80 g baby spinach

1 tablespoon lime juice

2 teaspoons extra-virgin olive oil

2 tablespoons coarsely chopped
  parsley

freshly cracked black pepper

¼ cup coarsely chopped walnuts

1. Combine the pears, spinach, lime juice, oil and half the parsley in a large bowl. Season and gently toss to coat.

2. Sprinkle with the walnuts and remaining parsley.

TIPS

- Pears oxidise and turn brown when cut. Adding an acid, like lime juice, prevents this from happening, so make sure you've squeezed your lime before slicing your pears.

- Try adding 125 g smoked chicken for a main meal (349 calories per serve).

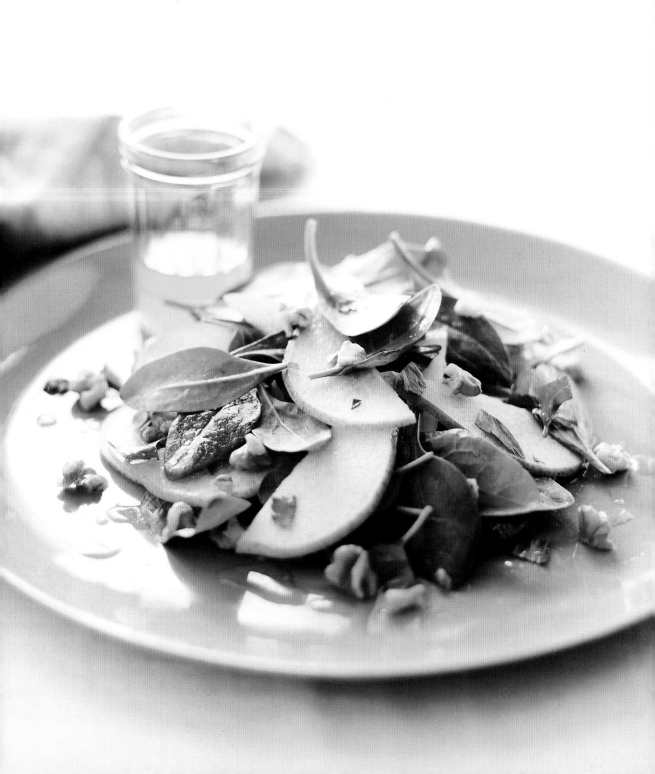

Watercress, fetta and watermelon salad

This is one of those salads that you eat visually before tasting. It looks so amazing on the table. Everyone will want to try it, and once they do it will become an instant favourite.

Serves 2

Prep 15 minutes

247 cal per serve

1 bunch watercress, trimmed and
   leaves picked

¼ cup torn mint leaves

¼ small red onion, thinly sliced

1 tablespoon white wine vinegar

2 teaspoons extra virgin olive oil

freshly cracked black pepper

800 g watermelon, peeled and cut
   into small wedges

100 g low-cal fetta, crumbled

1. Combine the watercress, mint, onion, vinegar and oil in a bowl. Season.

2. Toss to coat and transfer to a large plate. Top with the watermelon and fetta.

TIPS

- Watercress grows in water and doesn't survive long in the fridge, so try to buy it on the day you'll be using it.

- Keep mint wrapped in a damp cloth in the fridge. If it has gone limp, soak it in cold water for 15 minutes and drain before using.

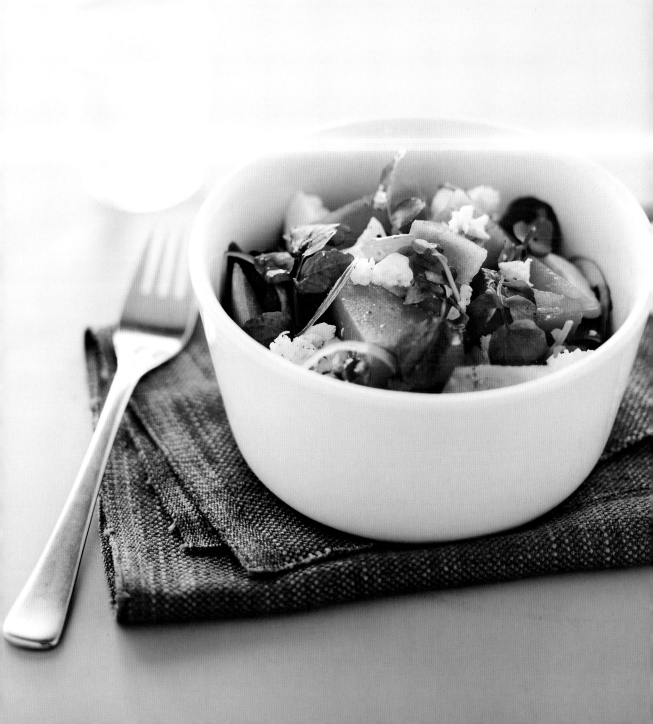

Cucumber, beetroot, chicken and mint salad

I love this satisfying chicken salad. The combination of chicken and chickpeas fills you up, and the mix of beetroot, red wine vinegar and mint kicks in mouth-watering flavours.

Serves 2
Prep 15 minutes
Cook 10 minutes
259 cal per serve

125 g chicken breast fillet, trimmed
freshly cracked black pepper
olive oil spray
1 small cucumber, halved lengthways
    and thinly sliced
125 g can chickpeas, drained
    and rinsed

70 g baby rocket
¼ cup coarsely chopped mint
1 tablespoon red wine vinegar
2 teaspoons extra virgin olive oil
½ clove garlic, crushed
440 g can baby beets, drained
    and halved or quartered

1. Season the chicken with pepper.

2. Spray a small non-stick frying pan with oil and heat on medium–high. Cook the chicken for about 8 minutes or until cooked through and browned. Slice the chicken.

3. Meanwhile, combine the cucumber, chickpeas, rocket and 2 tablespoons of the mint in a salad bowl. Make a dressing by combining the vinegar, oil and garlic in a small bowl. Season.

4. Drizzle the salad with the dressing and gently toss to coat. Top with the chicken and beetroot. Sprinkle with the remaining mint.

TIPS

- Use plastic gloves to handle the beetroot or your hands will be stained purple. Similarly, if you add the beetroot to the salad before tossing through the dressing, the purple juices tend to colour the whole salad.

- To keep the chicken breast moist, avoid cooking it over a very high heat; slower and longer will give you a better result.

- You can also add 300 g freshly cooked beetroot and 80 g home-cooked chickpeas (you'll need to cook 35 g of dried peas).

- For a vegetarian variation, omit the chicken and add 400 g canned chickpeas (254 calories per serve).

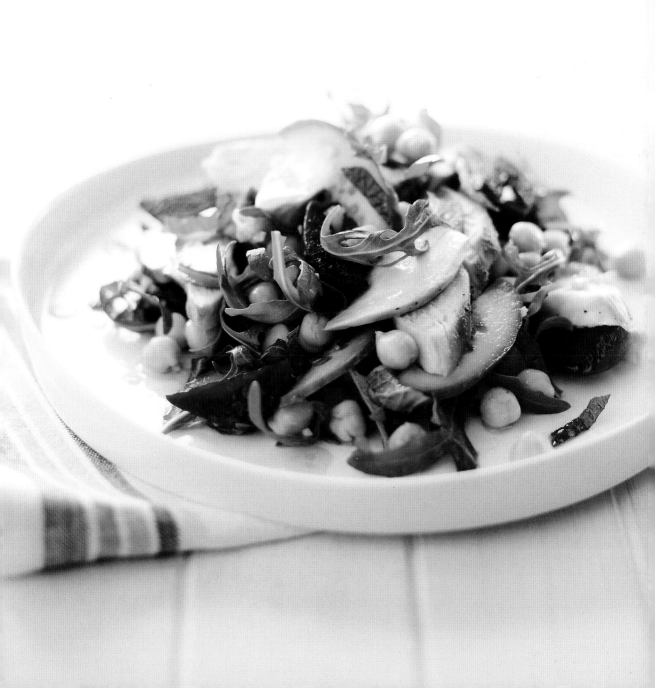

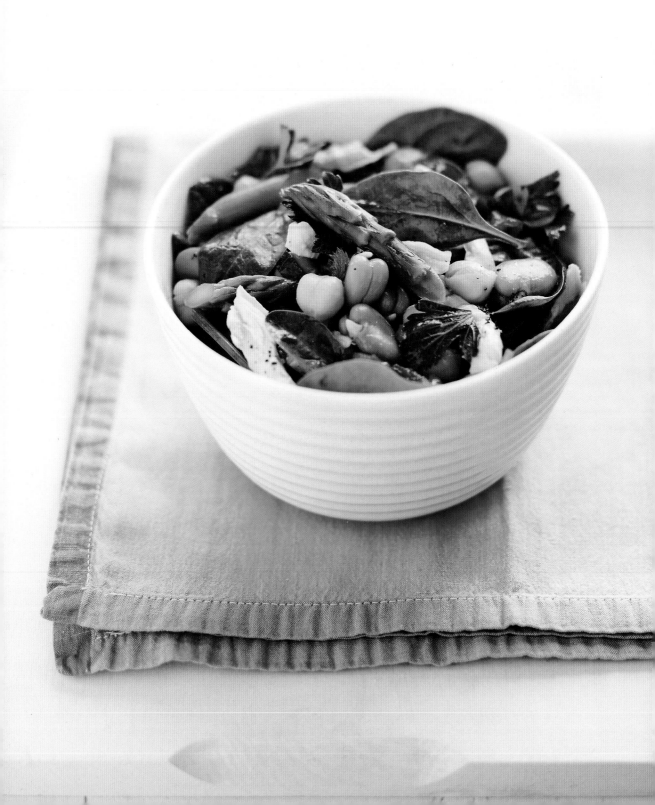

Poached chicken, broad bean, chickpea and sundried tomato salad

Poached chicken has changed my life – never again will I gag on a piece of dry chicken breast! In fact, this recipe ticks all the boxes: it's fast, low in calories, high in protein and delicious. The legume salad has a great chew to it, and it leaves me feeling satisfied.

180 g chicken breast fillet
1 cup frozen broad beans
1 bunch asparagus, trimmed
   and cut into chunks
125 g can chickpeas, drained
   and rinsed
70 g baby spinach

30 g sundried tomatoes, sliced
1 tablespoon red wine vinegar
2 teaspoons extra virgin olive oil
freshly cracked black pepper
2 tablespoons coarsely chopped
   parsley

Serves 2
Prep 15 minutes
Cook 15 minutes
302 cal per serve

1. Place the chicken in a small saucepan and cover with water. Bring to the boil. Reduce the heat and simmer for 4 minutes. Remove the pan from the heat and leave the chicken in the cooking liquid for 10 minutes to cook through. Remove the chicken from the liquid.

2. When cool enough to handle, shred the chicken. Cool the chicken stock and refrigerate or freeze for another use.

3. Cook the broad beans and asparagus in a saucepan of lightly salted boiling water for 2 minutes. Drain and refresh in cold water. Drain again.

4. Peel the broad beans and discard the skins.

5. Combine the broad beans, asparagus, chickpeas, spinach, tomato and chicken in a salad bowl. Make a dressing by combining the vinegar and oil in a small bowl. Season with pepper.

6. Drizzle the dressing over the salad and toss to coat. Sprinkle with parsley.

TIPS

● Broad beans are a pain to peel but it's worth the effort when you see their bright-green colour and taste them.

Pepper-crusted tuna with curly endive and cherry tomatoes

Tuna does not get any better than this. It looks beautiful on the plate, and it is the kind of meal that will have those last five kilos melting away. Love it!

Serves 2
Prep 15 minutes
Cook 15 minutes
291 cal per serve

1 bunch asparagus, trimmed
80 g curly endive
200 g cherry tomatoes, halved
1 tablespoon lemon juice

3 teaspoons extra virgin olive oil
freshly cracked black pepper
250 g fresh tuna
2 tablespoons torn basil leaves

1. Cook the asparagus in a small saucepan of lightly salted boiling water for 1 minute. Drain and cool in iced water. Drain again.

2. Combine the endive, tomatoes and asparagus in a salad bowl. Make a dressing by combining the lemon juice and 2 teaspoons of the oil in a small bowl. Season.

3. Coat the tuna with a little pepper. Heat the remaining oil in a non-stick frying pan and cook the tuna for 2 minutes until seared but still pink inside. Cut into strips.

4. Drizzle the dressing over the salad and toss to coat. Serve topped with the tuna and basil.

TIPS

- Don't overcook the tuna or it will be dry.
- Choose lighter endive leaves (the heart), as the dark leaves are very bitter.

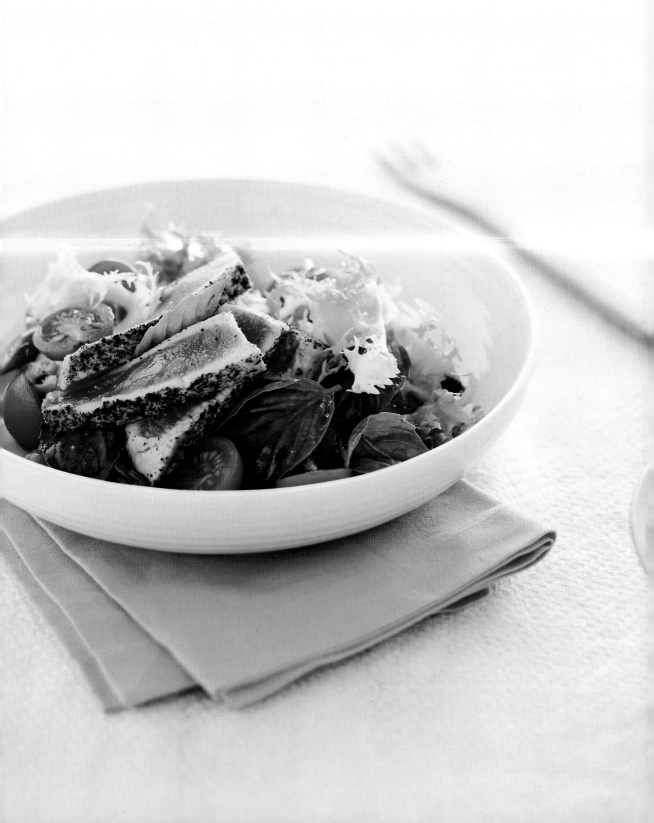

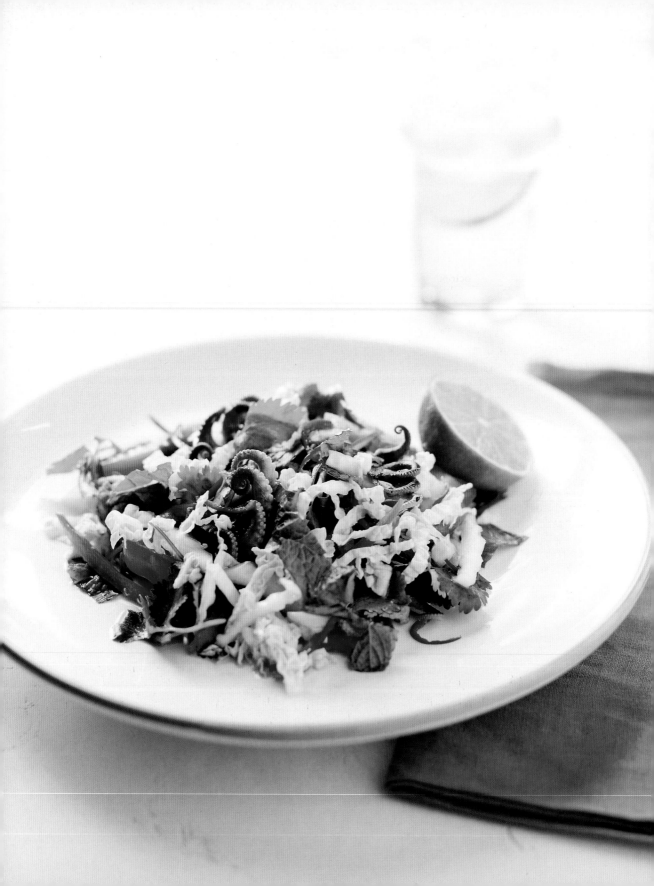

Thai octopus salad

Far from just boring lettuce leaves and some token tomatoes, salads can be whatever your imagination allows. This Thai octopus salad is a total winner. The flavours are crisp and fresh, and as well as having great texture it looks amazing. It's a summer essential!

300 g cleaned baby octopus,
    cut into chunks
¼ cup lime juice
1 clove garlic, thinly sliced
freshly cracked black pepper
2 teaspoons fish sauce
2 teaspoons brown sugar

1 long red chilli, finely chopped
cooking oil spray
250 g wombok, shredded
200 g baby roma tomatoes, halved
1 small red capsicum, thinly sliced
½ cup coriander leaves
¼ cup torn mint leaves

Serves 2
Prep 20 minutes
Cook 10 minutes
247 cal per serve

1. Combine the octopus, 1 tablespoon of the lime juice and the garlic in a bowl. Season with pepper.

2. Make a dressing by combining the remaining lime juice with the fish sauce, sugar and chilli in a small bowl.

3. Spray a char-grill pan with oil and heat on medium. Cook the drained octopus until tender and lightly charred.

4. Combine the wombok, tomatoes, capsicum and herbs in a salad bowl. Drizzle over the dressing and gently toss to coat. Serve topped with the octopus.

TIPS

- Ask your fishmonger to clean the baby octopus. If it hasn't been done, remove the beak, slit the head open and remove the ink sac. Rinse and pat dry with paper towel.

- The trick is not to overcook the octopus, as it tends to toughen. The point to look out for is when it changes colour. If you're unsure, cut a small piece to try it.

- Instead of octopus, you can make this salad with 250 g chicken breast (245 calories per serve) or 500 g rump steak (237 calories per serve).

Scallop, fennel and grapefruit salad

I have to say, I get excited when I know my husband is going to make this dish. The flavours are so clean and refreshing. It is his speciality, and we often have it for lunch on a Sunday while reading the papers. Heaven!

Serves 2
Prep 15 minutes
Cook 10 minutes
255 cal per serve

200 g fennel, trimmed
  and thinly sliced
70 g wild rocket
3 red radishes, thinly sliced
1 tablespoon white wine vinegar

2 teaspoons extra virgin olive oil
freshly cracked black pepper
1 large pink grapefruit, segmented
1 teaspoon olive oil
350 g scallops

1. Combine the fennel, rocket, radish, vinegar and extra virgin olive oil in a bowl. Season with pepper and toss to coat.

2. Transfer to a large plate and top with the grapefruit.

3. Heat the olive oil in a large non-stick frying pan on high. Cook the scallops for 1–2 minutes on each side until golden.

4. Top the salad with the scallops.

TIPS

- Look for fresh scallops, as frozen scallops release a lot of liquid when they cook and you end up stewing them.

- Segment the grapefruit over a bowl and enjoy the juice, but don't add it to the salad or you'll drown the fennel and rocket.

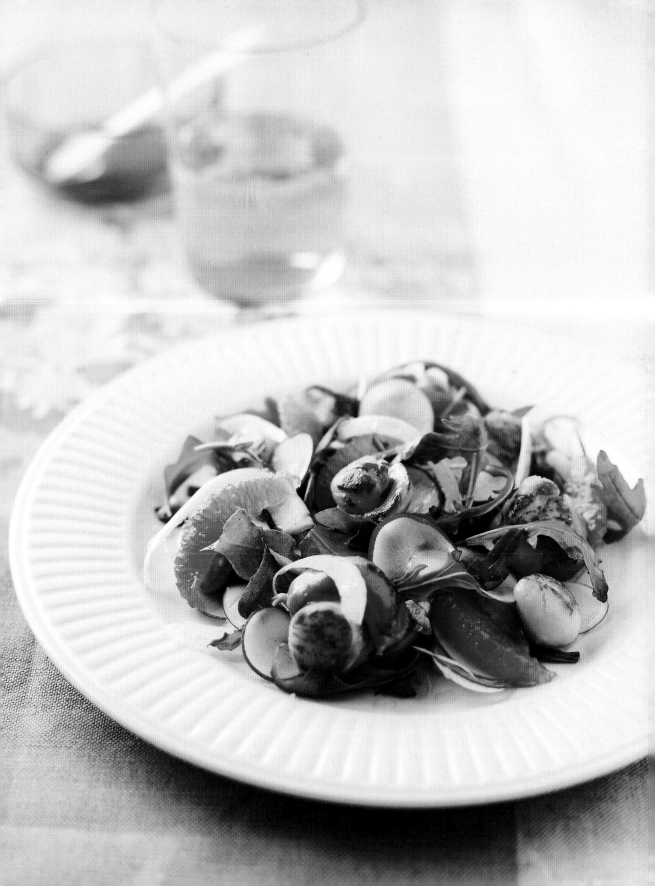

Spiced chargrilled vegetables with minted cracked wheat

The spices make all the difference to these veggies – they look fantastic, smell like heaven and taste delicious. Cracked wheat will cook faster if you soak it. You can serve it al dente with a slight crunch or softer, according to taste.

Serves 2
Prep 10 minutes
Cook 25 minutes
281 cal per serve

1 cup cracked wheat
250 ml salt-reduced vegetable stock
250 ml water
¼ cup finely chopped mint
1 small eggplant, thickly sliced
1 large zucchini, thickly sliced
1 tablespoon ras el hanout spice mix

olive oil spray
1 red capsicum, halved
½ cup low-cal yoghurt
¼ cup finely chopped coriander
2 teaspoons lemon juice
freshly cracked black pepper

1. Combine the cracked wheat, stock and water in a saucepan. Bring to the boil. Reduce the heat and simmer for 20–25 minutes or until al dente. Stir in the mint.

2. Meanwhile, steam the eggplant for about 10 minutes or until nearly cooked.

3. Sprinkle the zucchini with half the ras el hanout spice mix. Spray a char-grill pan with oil and heat on medium–high. Cook the zucchini and capsicum until tender and lightly charred.

4. Sprinkle the remaining spice mix over the eggplant and char-grill until lightly charred.

5. Combine the yoghurt, coriander and lemon juice in a small bowl. Season with pepper.

6. Cut the capsicum and eggplant into strips. Serve the cracked wheat with the vegetables and a dollop of yoghurt mixture.

TIPS

- Ras el hanout is a spice mix used in Morocco for tagines and kebabs. You can use it as a dry rub for meat and fish.

- Eggplants just love oil and tend to need a lot of it to cook. Steaming the eggplant before you chargrill it helps to reduce the amount of oil you need.

- If you prefer couscous instead of cracked wheat, combine ½ cup couscous and 125 ml boiling water in a bowl. Stand, covered, for 5 minutes, then fluff it up with a fork and stir through 2 tablespoons mint (338 calories per serve).

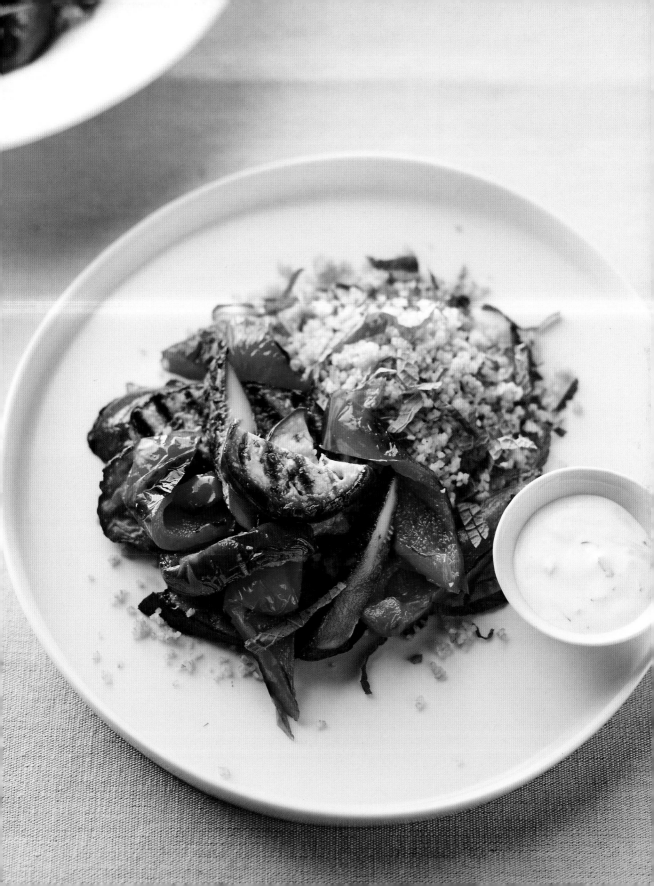

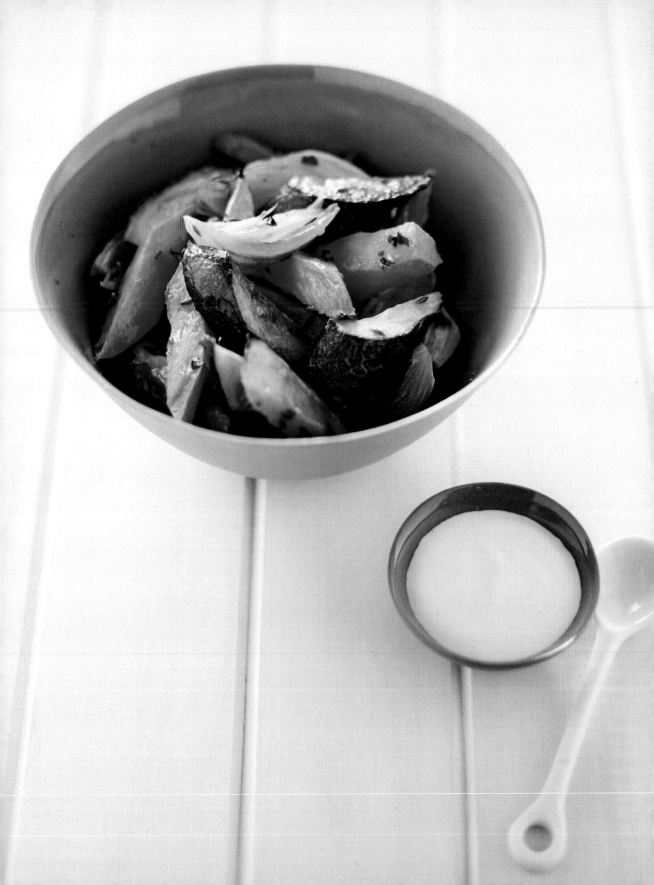

Cumin and chilli roasted vegetables with roasted garlic yoghurt

This dish has great wow factor for dinner parties. How could you not love vegetables when they are cooked this way? Once you try the garlic yogurt you will really be blown away.

550 g pumpkin, unpeeled, seeded and cut into 4 cm chunks

2 onions, quartered

1 large zucchini, cut into 4 cm chunks

1 large carrot, cut into 4 cm chunks

½ lemon, quartered

6 cloves garlic, unpeeled

2 teaspoons cumin seeds

¼ teaspoon dried chilli flakes

freshly cracked black pepper

2 teaspoons olive oil

½ cup low-cal yoghurt

Serves 2
Prep 10 minutes
Cook 30 minutes
287 cal per serve

1. Preheat the oven to 200°C/180°C fan-forced.

2. Combine the vegetables and garlic in a large baking dish. Sprinkle with the cumin and chilli and season with pepper. Drizzle with the oil and toss to coat.

3. Roast the vegetables for 30 minutes, stirring after 15 minutes.

4. Remove the garlic from the baking dish and squeeze out the flesh. Combine with the yoghurt and season.

5. Serve the roasted vegetables with the roasted garlic yoghurt and a lemon quarter to sqeeze on top.

TIPS

- Use a baking dish that is large enough to fit all the vegetables in a single layer.
- Make sure the chunks of vegetables are roughly the same size, so they cook evenly.
- These vegetables go really well with kangaroo fillet. Halve the amount of pumpkin and onion and pan-fry 200 g kangaroo while the vegetables are roasting (309 calories per serve).

Cauliflower and celeriac Madras curry

What a clever way to enjoy your veggies and satisfy your love for curry, all at the same time. You can use 1 tablespoon of a ready-made Madras curry paste instead of the garlic, ginger and spices (322 calories per serve).

Serves 2

Prep 10 minutes

Cook 40 minutes

269 cal per serve

2 tablespoons tomato paste

375 ml cups water

cooking oil spray

1 onion, thinly sliced

2 cloves garlic, crushed

1 tablespoon finely grated ginger

1 tablespoon ground coriander

2 teaspoons ground cumin

½ teaspoon turmeric

¼ teaspoon chilli powder

½ cup low-cal yoghurt

800 g celeriac, trimmed, peeled
and cut into chunks

freshly cracked black pepper

500 g cauliflower, broken into florets

¼ cup coriander leaves

2 tablespoons roasted slivered
almonds

1. Combine the tomato paste and water in a jug.

2. Spray a large saucepan with oil and heat on medium. Add the onion and cook, stirring occasionally, for 8 minutes until soft.

3. Stir in the garlic, ginger and spices and cook until fragrant.

4. Add the yoghurt and stir to combine. Stir in the diluted tomato paste. Add the celeriac and stir to coat. Season with pepper.

5. Bring to a gentle simmer and cook, covered, for 15 minutes. Stir in the cauliflower and cook, covered, for another 15 minutes.

6. Scatter the curry with the coriander and almonds to serve.

TIPS

- It's best to dilute tomato paste in water or stock before adding it to curries or stews to prevent it from burning on the bottom of the pan.

- For a Madras chicken curry, cut back the amount of celeriac and cauliflower by a quarter and stir through 125 g sliced chicken breast at the end.

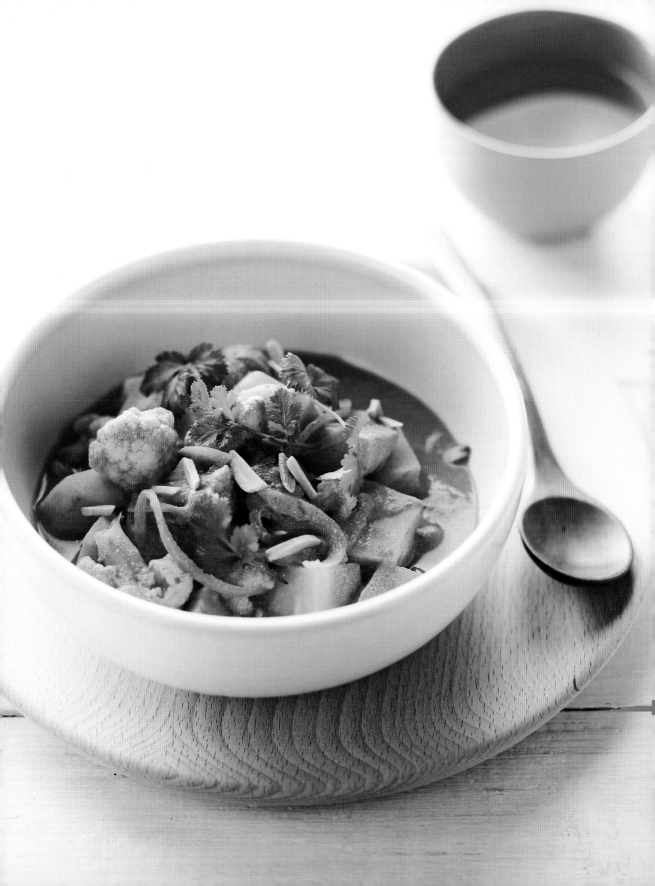

Stir-fried choy sum with chicken and soba noodles

Stir-fries are a staple on my dinner table – we have at least one a week. By using interesting flavours you can create something very special. Soba noodles will have you feeling full and they have a great 'chew' factor.

Serves 2
Prep 15 minutes
Cook 10 minutes
293 cal per serve

750 g choy sum
100 g dried soba noodles
cooking oil spray
80 g chicken breast fillet,
   sliced into thin strips

3 cloves garlic, crushed
1 tablespoon finely grated ginger
1 long red chilli, thinly sliced
2 teaspoons lime juice
1 teaspoon fish sauce

1. Slice the choy sum stems and set aside. Coarsely chop the leaves and set aside.

2. Cook the noodles in a small saucepan of boiling water for 3 minutes. Drain and rinse under cold water. Drain again.

3. Spray a wok with oil and heat on high. Stir-fry the chicken until browned and cooked through. Remove from the wok and set aside.

4. Respray the wok with oil. Stir-fry the choy sum stems, garlic, ginger and chilli until just tender.

5. Return the chicken to the wok with the noodles and gently stir-fry until heated through. Add the choy sum leaves, lime juice and fish sauce, and stir-fry until the leaves are just wilted. Serve immediately.

TIPS

- Soba noodles are made from buckwheat. Sold dried, you'll find them in the Asian section of supermarkets. You can also use them in soups and salads.

- For a vegetarian stir-fry, omit the chicken and increase the noodles to 130 g (292 calories per serve). You can find vegetarian fish sauce in Vietnamese stores.

- Take care not to overcook the choy sum.

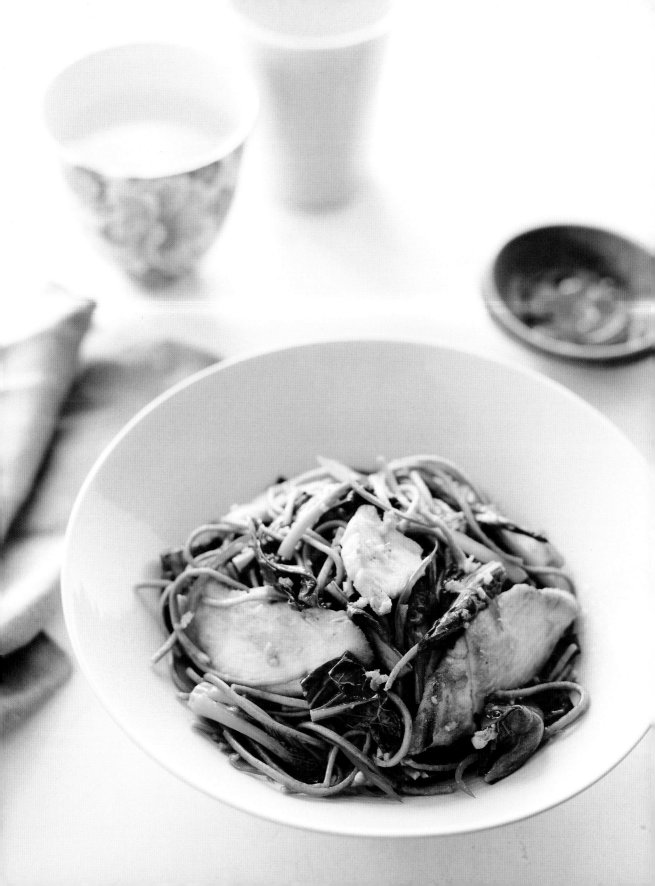

Pan-fried chicken with steamed Asian greens

This dish is the ultimate busy person's dinner. It's super high in vitamins, perfectly low in fat and a great source of protein. Best of all, it takes less time to cook than ordering take-away, and it's way cheaper too. I love big flavours, so the ginger is perfect.

Serves 2
Prep 15 minutes
Cook 10 minutes
303 cal per serve

cooking oil spray
2 × 150 g chicken breast fillets, trimmed
2 cloves garlic, thickly sliced
2 cm piece fresh ginger, shredded
1 bunch baby bok choy

1 bunch broccolini, trimmed
2 shallots, finely shredded
1 tablespoon oyster sauce
1 teaspoon soy sauce
1 teaspoon water
2 tablespoons coriander sprigs

1. Spray a non-stick frying pan with oil and heat on medium–high. Cook the chicken for about 8 minutes or until browned and cooked through.

2. Meanwhile, scatter the garlic and ginger in a steamer. Top with the bok choy and broccolini and scatter over the shallot. Steam, covered, over a large frying pan of simmering water for 6–8 minutes or until cooked to your liking.

3. Heat the oyster sauce, soy sauce and water in a small saucepan.

4. Top the chicken with the garlic, ginger, shallot and coriander sprigs. Drizzle over the sauce and serve with the steamed bok choy and broccolini.

TIPS

- You will often find grit lodged in between baby bok choy leaves, so take the time to soak and rinse the bulbs.

- You could steam the chicken for 8–10 minutes instead of pan-frying it.

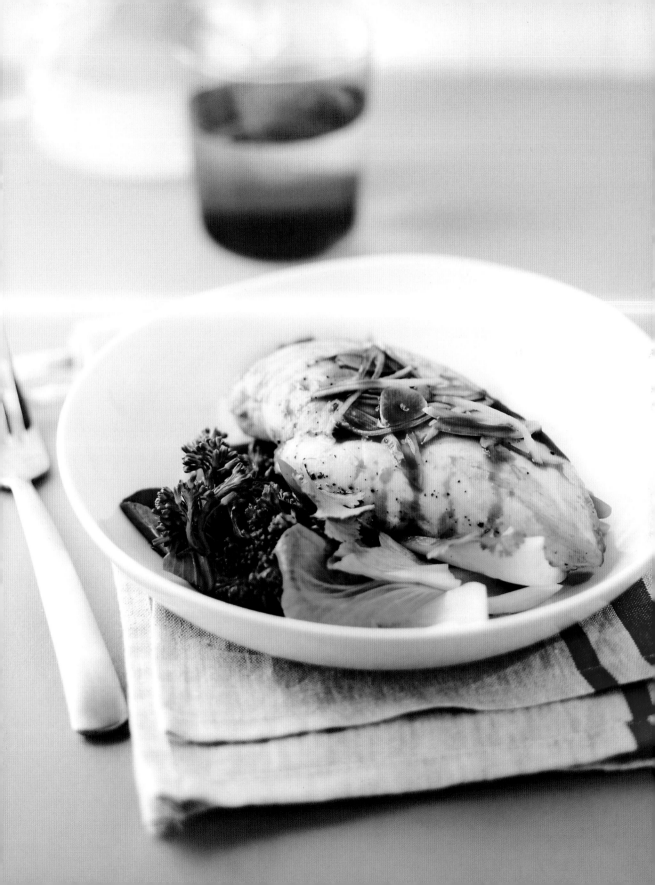

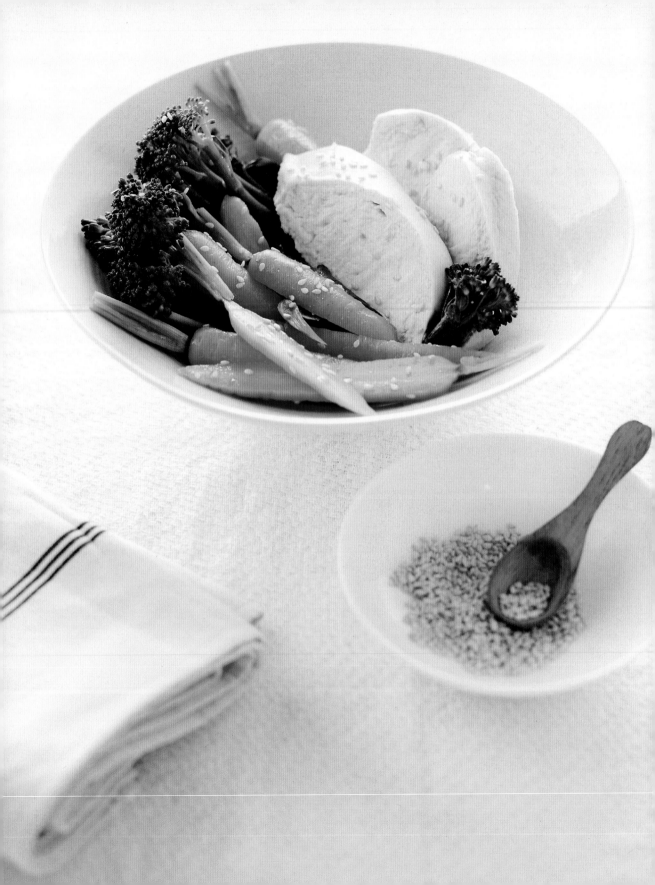

Steamed minted chicken with broccolini and baby carrots

This moist, mint-flavoured chicken takes just 10 minutes to cook. It proves you can whip up a stylish and healthy meal in no time flat. If you're cooking for one, use the other serving for lunch the next day.

2 mint sprigs
200 g chicken breast fillet
freshly cracked black pepper
1 bunch baby carrots, trimmed
1 bunch broccolini

2 teaspoons extra virgin olive oil
1 tablespoon toasted white
   sesame seeds

Serves 2
Prep 10 minutes
Cook 10 minutes
279 cal per serve

1. Place the mint sprigs in a large steamer, reserving several leaves, and top with the chicken. Season with pepper and scatter with the reserved mint leaves. Place the carrots next to the chicken. Steam, covered, over a large frying pan of simmering water for 5 minutes.

2. Add the broccolini and steam for another 5 minutes or until the chicken is cooked through.

3. Drizzle the vegetables with the oil and sprinkle with the sesame seeds. Slice the chicken and serve with the vegetables.

TIPS

- Steaming is a wonderful way of cooking, infusing the flavours and keeping the meat moist.

- You can vary the vegetables and herbs. Try steaming a fillet of salmon with sliced tomato and thyme, and sliced zucchini.

Stir-fried snapper with asparagus, wombok and shiitake mushrooms

This is definitely one of my all-time favourite stir-fries. The flavours are fresh and clean, and it will have you slipping back into your old jeans in no time!

Serves 2
Prep 15 minutes
Cook 15 minutes
260 cal per serve

300 g snapper fillet, skinned and
   cut into cubes
2 cloves garlic, crushed
1 tablespoon finely grated ginger
2 teaspoons salt-reduced soy sauce
cooking oil spray

1 bunch asparagus, cut into chunks
200 g shiitake mushrooms, sliced
3 shallots, finely sliced
300 g wombok, finely shredded
2 tablespoons oyster sauce
1 long red chilli, shredded

1. Combine the snapper, garlic, ginger and soy sauce in a bowl.

2. Spray a non-stick wok with oil and heat on medium. Stir-fry the fish for a few minutes until cooked. Remove from the wok.

3. Respray the wok with oil. Stir-fry the asparagus for 2 minutes. Add the mushrooms and half the shallot and stir-fry for 3–4 minutes or until tender. Add the wombok and oyster sauce and stir-fry until just wilted. Return the fish to the wok and gently toss through.

4. Serve the fish sprinkled with the remaining shallot and chilli.

TIPS

- When you're cooking with only a little oil, it's easier to use a non-stick pan or wok.

- Wombok releases a lot of liquid when it cooks, so only stir-fry it until it's just starting to wilt. The heat will continue to cook it.

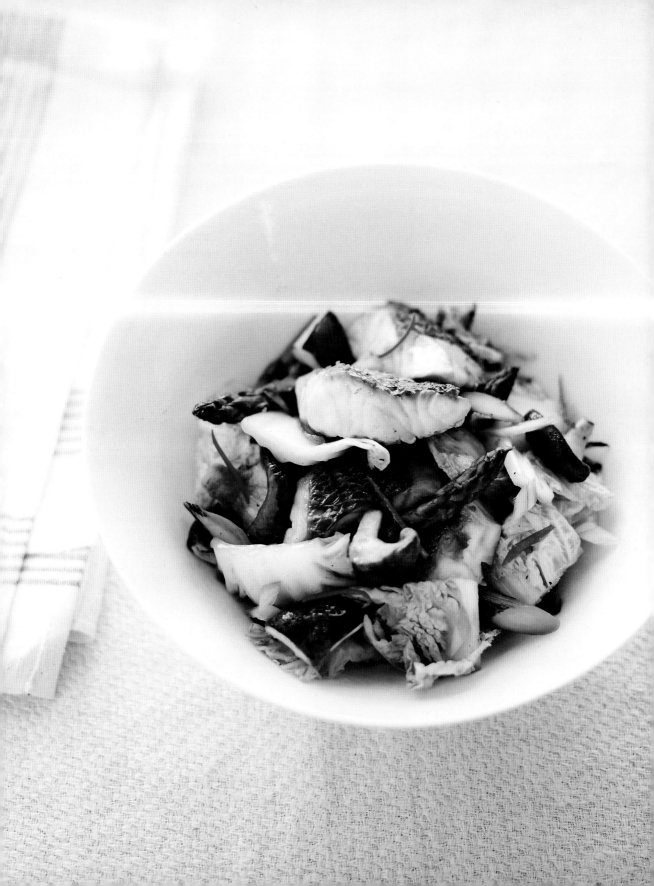

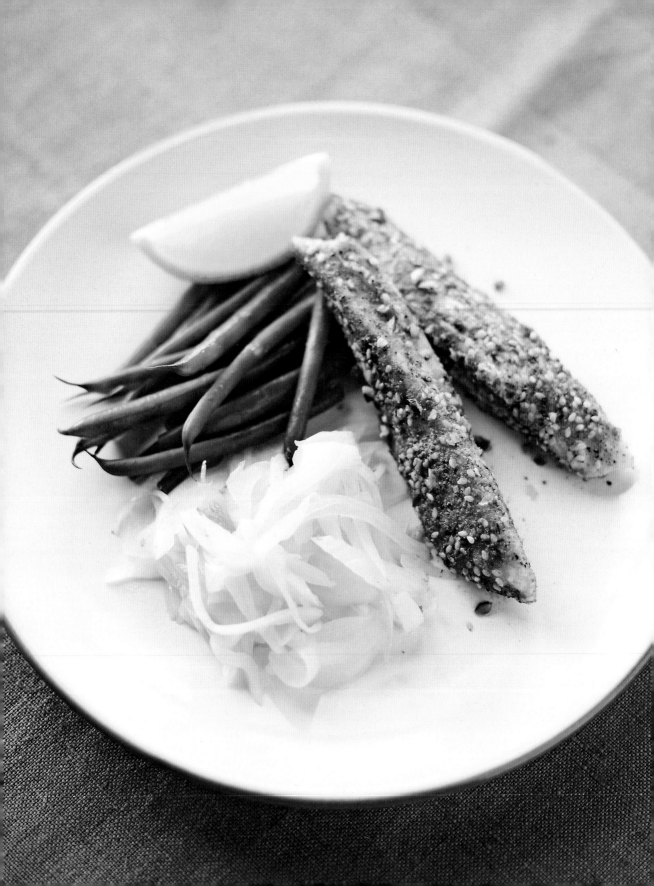

Dukkah-crusted flathead fillets with braised fennel and lemon

Dukkah is the new black! It really is quite marvellous when it comes to introducing new flavours. We love it on all kinds of fish, but flathead is definitely our favourite. I adore fennel, and braising it makes the flavour more subtle.

olive oil spray
400 g fennel, trimmed and
    thinly sliced
finely shredded zest of ½ lemon
1 tablespoon lemon juice

80 ml water
freshly cracked black pepper
150 g small green beans, trimmed
350 g flathead fillets
2 tablespoons dukkah

Serves 2
Prep 10 minutes
Cook 20 minutes
274 cal per serve

1. Spray a saucepan with oil and heat on medium–high. Cook the fennel, stirring, for 2 minutes. Stir in the lemon zest, lemon juice and water. Season with pepper. Reduce the heat to low and cook, covered, for 15 minutes or until tender.

2. Meanwhile, cook the beans in a small saucepan of lightly salted boiling water for 4 minutes. Drain and return to the hot saucepan. Cover to keep warm.

3. Sprinkle the fish with the dukkah and season with pepper. Spray a non-stick frying pan with oil and heat on high. Cook the fish for 6–8 minutes or until cooked to your liking.

4. Serve the fish with the fennel and green beans.

TIPS

- Dukkah is made from a mix of ground nuts, spices and dried herbs. You will find several varieties in the spice section of your supermarket. In Middle Eastern countries it's traditionally used as a dip with bread and olive oil, but it does wonders sprinkled over vegetables and salads and used to coat lamb, chicken or fish. Beware though: 1 tablespoon is about 50 calories, so use it sparingly.

- You can also serve these fillets with a fennel salad. Combine sliced fennel with 2 tablespoons coarsely chopped parsley, 1 tablespoon white wine vinegar, 2 teaspoons extra virgin olive oil and 1 teaspoon rinsed and drained baby capers (295 calories per serve), and forget the green beans.

Oven-baked whole bream with garlic spinach

Fish is one of the best foods you can eat when it comes to good health and nutrition. If you are looking for super food, you've found it. Serving the fish whole can look quite dramatic too. The garlic spinach is amazing and will leave you feeling fantastic.

Serves 2
Prep 10 minutes
Cook 20 minutes
299 cal per serve

olive oil spray
½ lemon, sliced
4 cm piece ginger, shredded
½ bunch garlic chives, cut into
　6 cm lengths
550 g whole bream, gutted
　and scaled

freshly cracked black pepper
1 medium tomato, sliced
1 teaspoon olive oil
2 bunches spinach, washed
　and trimmed
2 cloves garlic, thinly sliced

1. Preheat the oven to 220°C/200°C fan-forced.

2. Spray a large baking dish with oil. Place half the lemon and ginger in the centre of the dish and top with the chives.

3. Season the fish inside and out with pepper. Place the remaining lemon and ginger and half the tomato in the fish cavity. Place the fish on top of the chives, and top with the remaining tomato.
   Bake for 20 minutes.

4. Meanwhile, heat the oil in a large non-stick frying pan on high. Cook the spinach and garlic, stirring, until the spinach is just wilted. Season.

5. Serve the fish with the garlic spinach.

TIPS

- You can easily double this recipe if you have guests.

- Garlic chives, also known as Chinese chives, have a very mild garlic flavour. You can add them to stir-fries or soups, and they are often used in Asian dumplings. You can find them in Asian supermarkets or large fruit and vegetable stores. If you can't find them, use shallots instead.

- Take the time to thoroughly wash the spinach, as it can often be gritty.

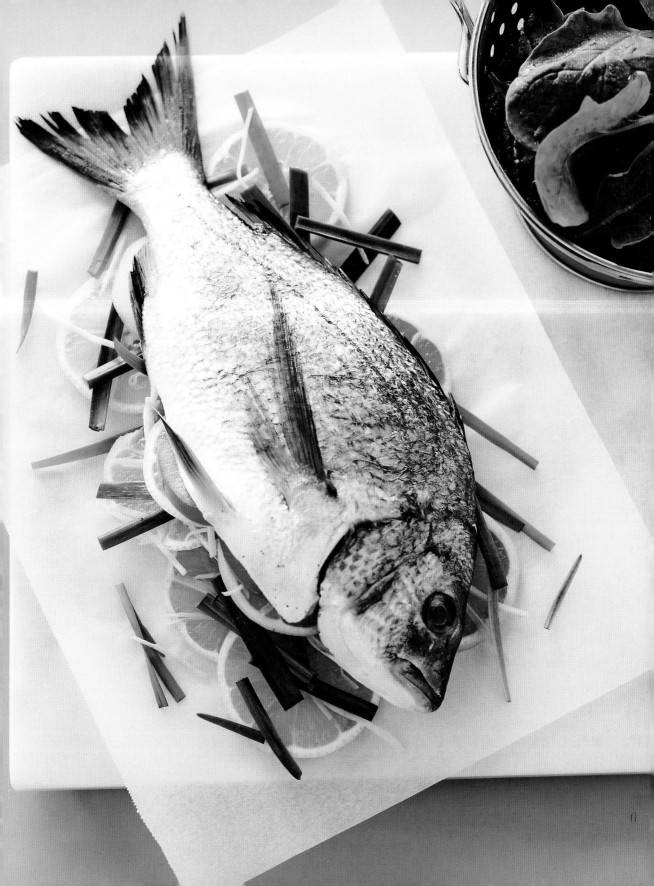

Chermoula prawn kebabs with couscous

These prawns have real wow factor. They are brilliant as an easy finger food for parties, and kids love to help make them. Couscous is a wonderful grain and works well with these flavours.

Serves 2

Prep 15 minutes

Marinate 20 minutes

Cook 5 minutes

301 cal per serve

1 shallot, finely chopped
½ teaspoon paprika
¼ teaspoon ground cumin
pinch of chilli powder
3–4 saffron threads
¼ cup chopped parsley
¼ cup chopped coriander
1 tablespoon lemon juice

450 g raw prawns, peeled, tailed
  and deveined
½ cup couscous
125 ml boiling water
freshly cracked black pepper
½ small cucumber, diced
2 tablespoons finely chopped mint
olive oil spray

1. To make the marinade, process the shallot, spices, parsley, coriander and lemon juice in a small blender. Combine the marinade and prawns in a shallow dish and turn to coat. Refrigerate, covered, for 20 minutes.

2. Meanwhile, stir the couscous into the boiling water. Season with pepper and stand, covered, for 5 minutes. Fluff up with a fork and stand for another 5 minutes. Stir through the cucumber and mint and season.

3. Spray a char-grill pan with oil and heat on high. Skewer the prawns onto 4 bamboo skewers. Cook the prawns for 2 minutes each side until pink and lightly charred.

4. Serve the prawns with the couscous.

TIPS

- You'll need about 20 medium prawns for this dish. You can leave the heads on or take them off.

- The marinade is also great for fish. Try it with 250 g snapper or flathead fillets (322 calories per serve).

- If you don't have a blender, simply chop all the marinade ingredients as finely as possible. You could use a garlic crusher to crush the finely chopped shallot.

- Soak the bamboo skewers in water for 30 minutes to prevent them from burning.

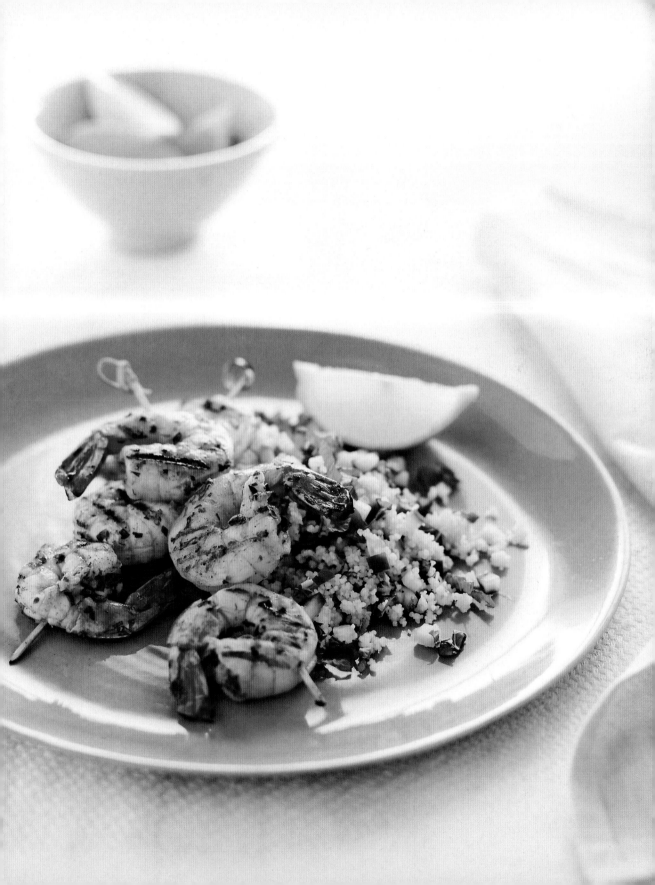

Beef fillet with coriander salsa

Quality over quantity is always my rule with beef. Add this amazing Cajun-style salsa to a great cut of meat, and you will be hailed as a master chef! This is food the whole family can enjoy, and it's dead easy to make. For hungry children and partners, add some brown rice or sweet potato to their plate.

Serves 2

Prep 15 minutes

Cook 10 minutes

302 cal per serve

1 corn cob

2 tomatoes, diced

1 small cucumber, diced

1 small green capsicum, diced

½ cup coriander leaves

2 teaspoons lemon juice

2 teaspoons extra virgin olive oil

1 clove garlic, crushed

freshly cracked black pepper

2 × 140 g beef fillets

1 tablespoon Cajun spice mix

olive oil spray

1. Cook the corn in a saucepan of salted boiling water for about 8 minutes or until tender. Drain and cut into 4 chunks.

2. Meanwhile, combine the tomato, cucumber, capsicum, coriander, lemon juice, oil and garlic in a bowl. Season with pepper and toss to coat.

3. Sprinkle the steaks with the spice mix. Spray a non-stick frying pan with oil and heat on high. Cook the steaks for 1–2 minutes each side for rare.

4. Serve the steaks with the salsa and corn on the cob.

TIPS

- If you like your meat rare, take it out of the fridge 15 minutes before cooking so the centre isn't cold. If you like it well done, it will take longer to cook so there is no need to take it out early.

- Cajun spice mix also goes well with fish and chicken. Next time you make this recipe, try using 300 g snapper fillet (268 calories per serve) or 250 g chicken breast (292 calories per serve).

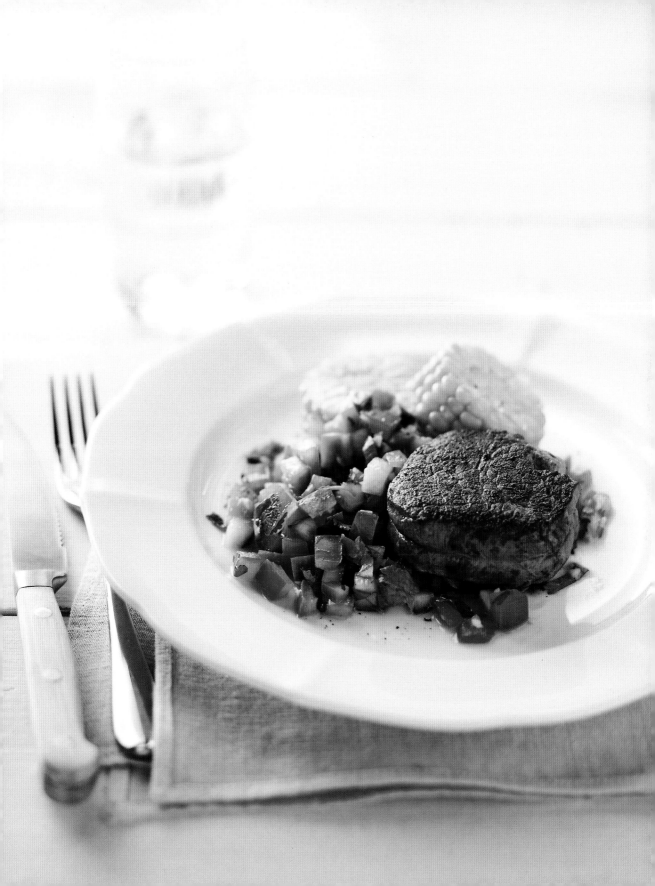

Kangaroo with grilled capsicum, cucumber, baby rocket and witlof salad

You want a super food? I give you kangaroo! Its properties will blow you away healthwise, and it's far better for the environment than cattle. The rich flavour of kangaroo leaves you feeling full and satisfied. Witlof is my new favourite salad ingredient – its great flavour brings a salad to life.

Serves 2
Prep 15 minutes
Cook 10 minutes
300 cal per serve

olive oil spray
1 red capsicum, halved and seeded
100 g canned butter beans,
  drained and rinsed
1 small cucumber, halved lengthways
  and sliced
50 g baby rocket

2 witlof, cored and thickly sliced
1 tablespoon white balsamic
  dressing
2 teaspoons extra virgin olive oil
300 g kangaroo fillet,
  cut into large chunks
freshly cracked black pepper

1. Spray a char-grill pan with oil. Cook the capsicum for about 5 minutes or until lightly charred and tender. Thickly slice the capsicum.

2. Combine the butter beans, cucumber, rocket, witlof and capsicum in a salad bowl. Place the balsamic dressing and oil in a small bowl and combine.

3. Season the kangaroo with pepper. Spray a non-stick frying pan with oil and heat on high. Cook the kangaroo for 1–2 minutes for rare. Remove from the heat and rest, loosely covered, for 5 minutes.

4. Drizzle the salad with the dressing and gently toss to coat. Serve with the kangaroo.

TIPS

- Witlof, or Belgian endive, is mildly bitter and crunchy. If you're not sure about the bitterness, choose the palest leaves and remove the centre core.

- Kangaroo is a very lean meat and tends to be tough if overcooked. Cut the fillet into large chunks and cook them in a very hot pan until well browned but still rare to medium–rare inside. Resting the meat allows it to relax and ensures greater tenderness.

- Instead of butter beans you could use 125 g canned chickpeas, drained and rinsed, or red kidney beans.

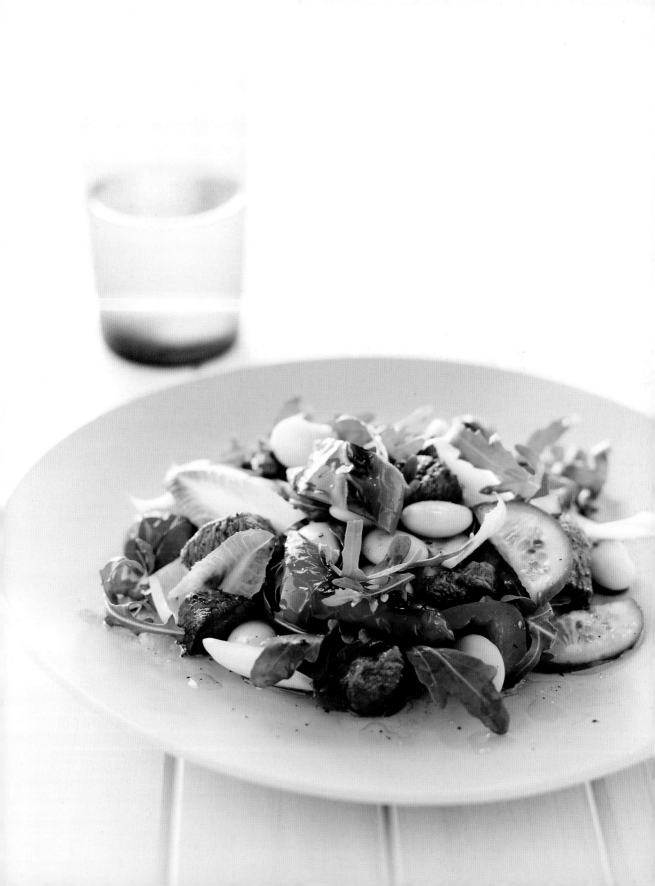

strength: upper body

push-ups (knees or toes)

1. Kneel on the ground and walk your hands forward until they are slightly wider than shoulder-width apart. Straighten your arms, keep your torso long and strong and look directly at the floor. Your knees can be hip-width apart or together.

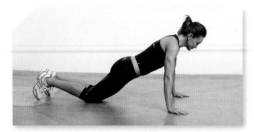

2. Keeping your abs pulled in, inhale, bend your elbows and lower your upper body until your chest is about 10 cms off the floor.

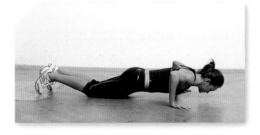

3. Try to keep your shoulders away from your ears as you exhale and straighten your arms to return to the start position.

variations
- Working on your toes is harder – avoid having your backside 'up'; think of your body as a long plank of wood.
- Try walking push-ups or having one hand on a low bench and then swapping.

fitball dumbbell chest press

1. Sit on the edge of the fitball and rest some light/medium dumbbells on your thighs. Walking your feet forward, roll down the fitball and lower your shoulders so that your body is horizontal.
2. Lift the dumbbells above your head, holding them approximately 10 cm apart with straight arms. Have your feet hip-width apart and squeeze your backside and thighs to keep you stable.

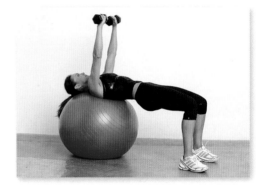

3. Keep your midsection braced and inhale as you lower the dumbbells towards the outside of your chest.

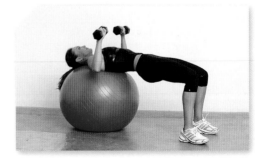

4. Exhale as you press the dumbbells back to the top.

triceps dips off a bench

1. Sit on a low bench and grip the edge with the heel of the hand on the bench, fingers wrapped around it. Support your weight through your arms and shoulders and walk your feet forward so that your thighs are parallel to the floor. The further out your feet, the harder it gets.
2. Inhale as you lower your body until your upper arms are almost horizontal to the floor. Avoid allowing your shoulders to scrunch up around your ears.
3. Exhale as you drive yourself up, squeezing the backs of your arms.

> *variation*
> - Try placing a weight in your lap for added intensity or having your feet up on a bench as well.

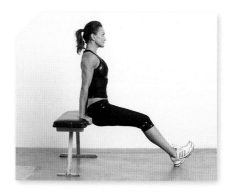

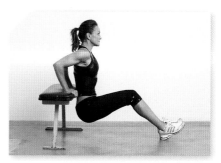

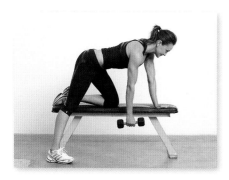

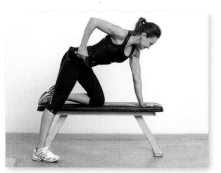

dumbbell rows

1. Select a medium/heavy dumbbell and place one knee on a bench. Support yourself by placing your free hand on the bench and your opposite foot slightly back and on the floor. Square up your shoulders and your hips and lock yourself into a strong position with a long straight spine. Allow the dumbbell to hang directly below your shoulder.
2. Exhale as you pull the dumbell up to your hip bone, keeping your elbow close to your torso. Avoid twisting through your body, stay still and strong.
3. Pause and inhale as you lower the dumbbell back to the starting position. Make sure to do both sides.

mountain climbers

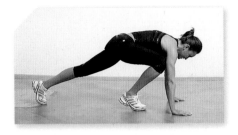

1. Start by kneeling on one knee and placing your hands either side of your front leg on the floor, slightly wider than your shoulders. Move your body weight forward onto your hands and lift the back knee up off the floor. You are now in start position.

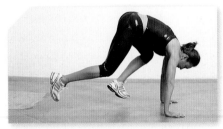

2. Spring both feet off the ground, switching position whilst most of your body weight is in your upper body. It's a relatively brisk switch back and forth.
3. Make sure to pull your abs in and stay strong through the shoulder and arms.

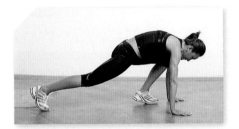

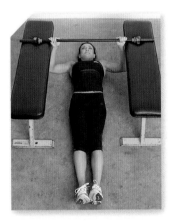

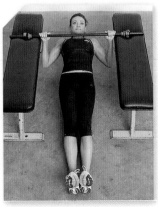

body rows

1. Lie on the floor underneath a secure bar placed across two benches. You can use a Smith machine in the gym for this as well.
2. Grip the bar slightly wider than shoulder width or more. Your body is long and now you must 'stiffen' it like a plank of wood, bracing your abs and squeezing your backside and thighs.
3. Exhale as you pull your chest toward the bar, squeezing your shoulder blades back and together. Inhale as you slowly lower yourself down. Avoid dropping completely to the floor – try to keep the tension on one rep after the other.

variation
- Using gym equipment like a Smith machine can help with heights of the bar. You can also have your feet elevated on a low bench.

standing dumbbell shoulder press

1. Holding light to medium dumbbells, stand tall with your feet in a split stance. Your front knee should be soft and take most of your weight; the ball of the back foot should be on the floor, your back leg acting as a prop to stop you from leaning backwards or arching your back. You should feel anchored into the ground, rock solid.

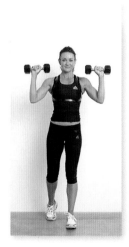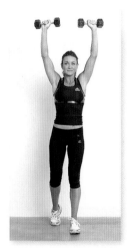

2. Keeping your midsection braced, exhale as you drive the dumbbells up, keeping them slightly forward of your face at the top of the movement. Do not lock out your elbows and do not push the dumbbells back behind your head.
3. Inhale as you carefully lower the dumbbells back to the start position. Make sure you maintain perfect posture throughout the movement.

variation
- Use a barbell

one-arm squat press

1. Holding a light to medium dumbbell in one hand, take your feet slightly wider than your hips, toes turned slightly out, centre of knee aligns with centre of your shoe. Place the other hand firmly on your hip and feel strong and braced within your core.

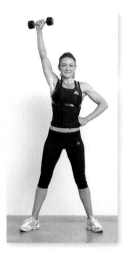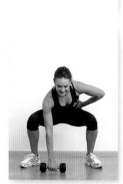

2. Bend your knees into a squat position and lean forward so as to tap your dumbbell to the floor. Be sure to maintain perfect posture, chest proud, shoulders back and down and abs pulled in.
3. Drive yourself up from the squat position and in the same motion pressing your dumbbell over your head once you get to standing position. Brace your core for extra drive to the top.

variation
- Try using kettle bells or do it with no weight and add a power jump in the air at the top.

strength: lower body

squat with barbell

1. Stand tall with your heels slightly wider than hip width apart and your feet slightly angled out. Place the barbell on the fleshy part of your upper back. Let the tension you feel between your shoulder blades help support the bar.

2. Inhale as you bend your legs and lower your hips until your thighs are just above parallel to the floor. The centre of your knee must align with the centre of your shoe as you move. Try to feel your weight in your heels, keep your chest proud and your back long, chin pulled in, rather than pushing it forward.

3. Exhale as you push through your heels and squeeze your butt to return to start position. Avoid locking out your knees at the top. Use a mirror to check your knees align with your toes.

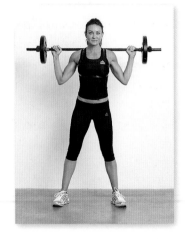

variation
- Mix up your rhythm by doing bottom half movements.

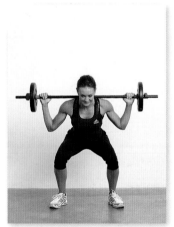

dumbbell fitball squats

1. Place a fitball between you and a solid wall so the ball is comfortably supporting your lower back. Step your feet forward and shoulder-width apart so that your heels are wider than your hips and your feet are slightly angled out. Let your arms hand by your sides holding two medium to heavy dumbbells.

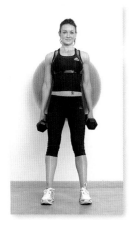 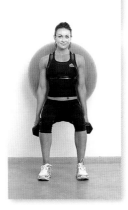

2. Inhale as you bend your legs, and lower your hips until your thighs are almost parallel to the floor. At the bottom of the movement your knees should not be sitting further forward of your toes. Because you are leaning up against the ball, your body will remain upright.

3. Exhale and push through your heels and squeeze your butt to return to the start position.

variations
- Do not use weights, take stance slightly wider or narrower; mix up the rhythm by doing bottom halves.

step-up with dumbbells

1. Use a bench knee height or lower and hold two medium to heavy dumbbells.

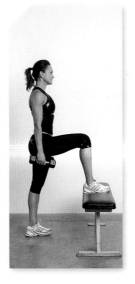 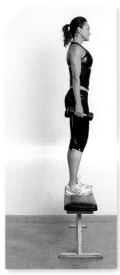

2. Step up onto the bench, maintaining a strong posture, long spine, chin in, shoulders back and down, abs pulled in.

3. Step down into the start position.

variation
- Try blowing out one leg completely by stepping up AND lowering down on the same leg. Use an 'up tap, down tap' rhythm and then swap.

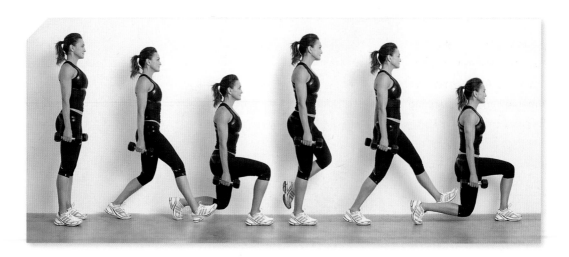

walking lunge with dumbbells

1. Holding medium dumbbells and maintaining a strong posture, step forward into a lunge position. Take a big step to avoid your knee pushing forward past your toes.

2. Look straight ahead and drop straight down rather than leaning forward or pushing the knee forward.

3. Push up using both legs and your butt and take your next step. Put some focus into pushing up 'through your front heel' so as to take pressure out of the knee. Avoid rushing; instead take your time to create two perfect right angles with both legs for every repetition.

> *variation*
> - Drop the weights and do it with body weight, or try holding a fitball out in front or above your head.

alternating backward dumbbell lunge

1. Standing with feet hip-width apart and holding two medium dumbbells. Imagine you are standing on two railway tracks. Inhale as you take a backwards step, sticking the ball of your foot to the floor where the track for that foot would be, and lowering yourself down 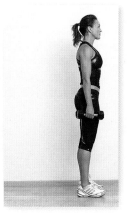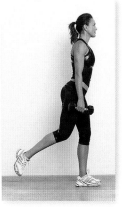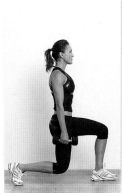 into a lunge. This stops you from wobbling around and losing your balance. Aim to create two perfect right angles with both legs.
2. Maintain strong posture, abs pulled in, chest proud, shoulders back and down, chin in as you drive up from the lunge back to the starting position.

variation
- Backwards lunges are the safest to do and a good starting point as they set you up in great technique. If you're new to lunges, lose the weights and hang onto a stable chair for a little support.

dynamic backward lunges on low step no dumbbells

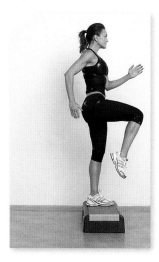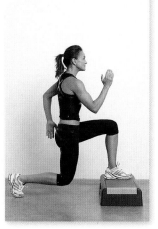

1. Standing feet-width apart on your low bench, imagine you are standing on two railway tracks. Inhale as you step back off the bench and down into a lunge, sticking the ball of the foot where the railway track would be. Aim to create two perfect right angles with both legs.
2. Maintain strong posture and using 'running' arms, powerfully drive yourself back up to the top, driving the knee through to the front.
3. Take the same leg back again. There are no weights with these, so step up the pace and get your heart rate flying.

cardio / agility / plyometric

fast low-step running

1. Using a low step, step up and down on your right leg and then swap for your left leg.
2. Keep this fast and pacey, maintaining strong posture throughout.

> *variation*
> - Try using a set of stairs. Go one step at a time, then try two steps at a time.

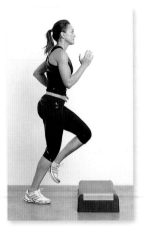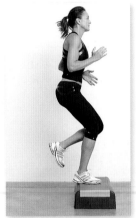

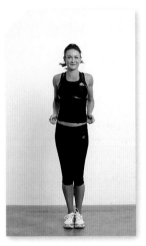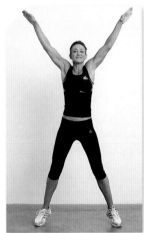

jumping jacks

1. Start with your feet together, pull in your abs, maintain strong posture and bend down into your legs.
2. Spring out with both feet landing into a shoulder-width-apart position, knees aligned with toes, knees like shock absorbers and arms stretched up and out.
3. Spring back into start position and repeat.

ice skaters

1. Lay a towel down on the ground or set up a low step platform and take a long, low leap over it, sideways.
2. Swing your arms in the direction you are travelling and land the foot solidly with the toes slighty pointed out, and the knee aligned with the toes.
3. As you land, sink deep into the leg to spring back across to the other side.

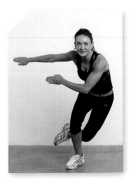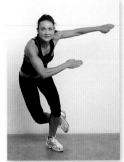

ski jumps

1. Keeping your toes and knees aligned and your knees soft like shock absorbers, switch on your abs and lift your chest.
2. Jump sideways over a line, towel or rope on the ground.
3. This is a spring-like action, so pump your arms to maintain your momentum.

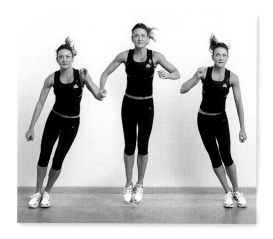

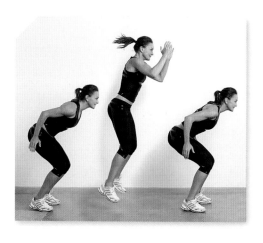

frog jumps

1. Start with your feet hip-width apart, abs pulled in, chest proud, shoulders back and down.
2. Sink deep into your legs as you swing both arms back behind you.
3. Swing your arms forward as you propel yourself forward and land softly, sinking straight back down into the legs. The jumps should flow, one after the other.

variation
- Try holding a medicine ball close to your chest to up the ante.

plyometric lunges

1. Start in a lunge postion and, using the power of your legs and the swing of your arms, spring up off the floor and swap legs.
2. Land into a perfect lunge and power straight up again.
3. These are pacey and should be done with momentum.

variation
- Try holding a medicine ball to up the ante.

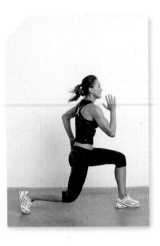 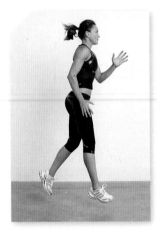 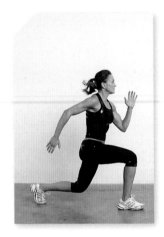

over the fence jumps

1. Standing beside a knee-high bench, place your hands firmly on either side of the bench.
2. With feet together, bend the knees and sink into your legs as you spring up and over the bench, landing softly with shock absorbers for legs.
3. Maintain your momentum and spring straight back to the original side. This is a pacey and energetic exercise.

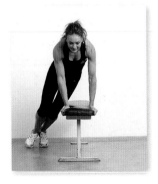 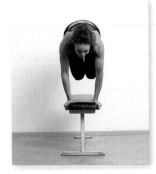 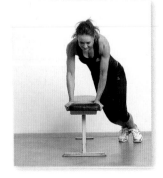

core: front & back

turkish get-up

1. Start by lying face up on the floor, holding a light dumbbell straight out in front of you.
2. Now begin to get yourself up off the floor without allowing the dumbbell to move from above your head.
3. Get all the way up to standing and then lower yourself back down to the start without allowing the dumbbell to drop.

variation
- These are tough, so try it without a weight but simply keep one arm up.

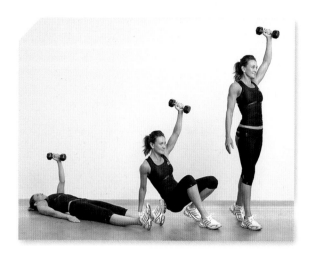

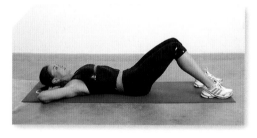

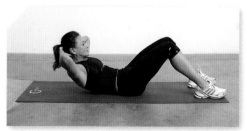

crunch

1. Lie on the floor and bend your knees so that your feet are flat on the floor. Draw your abs in, narrowing your waist and place your hands behind your head, keeping the elbows out of sight to avoid pulling on your head.
2. Keeping your abs tight, exhale as you roll or crunch up your upper torso. Keep your chin in and look forward.
3. Inhale and keep your abs drawn in as you lower yourself back down to the start postion. Avoid excessive back arch in the down phase – think pulling inwards.

variation
- Use a medicine ball.

double crunch

1. Lie on the floor and bend your knees so that your feet are flat on the floor. Draw your abs in, narrowing your waist and place your hands behind your head, keeping the elbows out of sight to avoid pulling on your head.

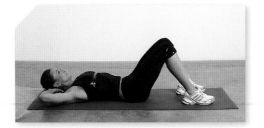

2. Keeping your abs tight, exhale as you roll or crunch up your upper torso whilst also drawing your knees towards your chest, lifting your butt just off the floor. Keep your chin in and look forward.

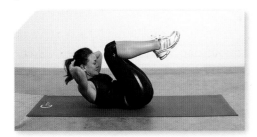

3. Inhale and keep your abs drawn in as you lower yourself back down to start position. Avoid excessive back arch in the down phase – think pulling inwards.

twisting crunch

1. Lie on the floor and bend your knees so that your feet are flat on the floor. Draw your abs in, narrowing your waist and place your hands behind your head, keeping the elbows out of sight to avoid pulling on your head.

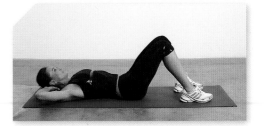

2. Keeping your abs tight, exhale as you lift and twist your shoulder across to the opposite knee.

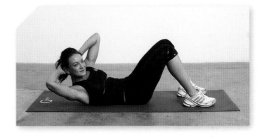

3. Inhale and keep your abs pulled in as you lower yourself back to the start position. Either stay focused on one side or alternate side to side.

variation
- Use a medicine ball if you are focusing on one side only, then swap.

lower body twist

1. Lie on the floor, lift your legs up and bend your knees to create a right angle. Place your arms directly out to the side, palms facing down, and squeeze your knees and ankles together so both legs are moving as one.

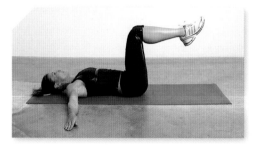

2. Inhale as you lower your legs down about halfway to one side, keeping your shoulders on the floor.

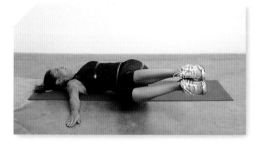

3. Exhale as you slowly drag the legs back to the centre and repeat on the other side.

variation

- Try squeezing a small medicine ball between your knees as you perform the movement.

single leg extension

1. Lie on your back and lift your legs above you, keeping your knees bent at 90 degrees and directly over your hips. Place your arms down beside you, palms down and keep your lower back firm against the floor. Now draw your belly button down into the floor and lock it in.

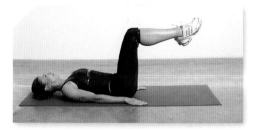

2. Keeping one leg in place, exhale and straighten the other leg away from you until you can no longer keep your abs pulled in. As soon as you feel your abs 'pop' outwards or your lower back starts to arch off the floor, you have extended too far for you. Pull your leg back until you can reset your abs inwards. The stronger you get, the further you will be able to extend your leg. Keep your head on the floor.

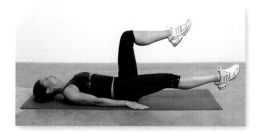

variation

- Once you get stronger, challenge yourself using all the above technique with two legs!

bicycle

1. Lie on your back and lift your legs above you, keeping your knees bent at 90 degrees and directly over your hips. Place your hands behind your head, with the elbows out of sight to avoid pulling on your head. Now draw your belly button down into the floor and lock it in.
2. Exhale as you lift up with a twisting action, bringing the shoulder towards the opposite knee and extend the other leg straight out.

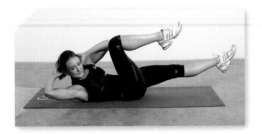

3. Inhale as the movement flows to the next side and exhale as you get the top of the twist.

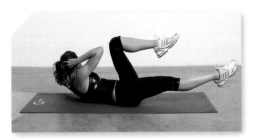

variation
- Try doing these on a Bosu ball – it really puts the pressure on.

plank (elbow)

1. Lay face down on the floor. Place your hands forward and flat, elbows directly under your shoulders. Lengthen your neck, pull your chin in and look at your hands. Keep your knees on the floor and hip-width apart. Your butt should be slightly lower than your shoulders and your body should feel like a strong plank of wood, so keep your abs pulled in.

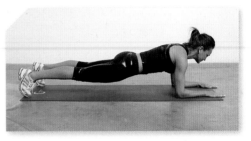

2. Get the feeling of pushing yourself away from the floor and to stabilize your shoulders, roll them back and away from your ears. Keep breathing steadily, keep your body in alignment and ever so slightly tuck your tailbone under.
3. When you are ready, push up onto your toes. Now your butt should be at the same level as your shoulders; your body all in one long line; perfect posture. Stay for as long as you can on your toes before going back to knees. Work your way up to 1 minute.

hand plank with twist

1. Lay face down on the floor, then push yourself up into a push-up position. Your hands should be about shoulder-width apart. Maintain perfect posture and alignment through your torso. Chin in, long neck, shoulders back and down, abs in and strong thighs.
2. Now turn onto one hand, opening your body up and into a side position. At the same time bring the same foot as the hand which is propping you up under and through, tapping it in front of you, forward on the floor.
3. Return your foot and hand to the start position and turn to the other side, now using the other arm and foot. You must maintain a strong and tight torso in order to move smoothly from one position to the next.

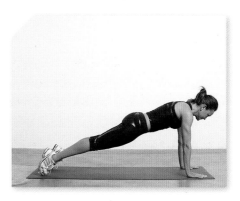

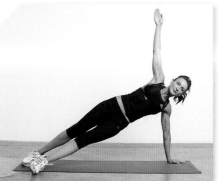

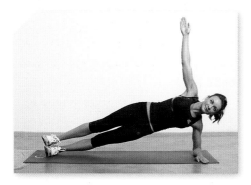

side plank (elbow) thread the needle

1. Lie on your side, raise yourself up on one elbow, palm flat, and 'stack' your shoulders, hips, knees and ankles, with feet perpendicular to the floor. Inhale as you open up your chest, stabilizing yourself on your elbow and hip. Push up 'out' of your shoulder and work from your knees to start with and move up onto your feet when you feel ready. It might take a few weeks.
2. Extend your other arm straight up to the roof to help you open your chest. Now bring the arm down and 'thread it' under you with a slight twist through the torso, then bring it back to the start position.
3. Maintain steady breathing whilst holding strong through your core and body.

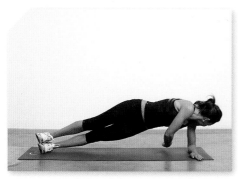

core: front & back   157

fitball crunch

1. Sit on the fitball and roll yourself down until your lower back and your thighs and torso are parallel with the floor. Draw your abs inwards, narrowing your waist and place your hand behind your head, keeping your elbows out of sight to avoid pulling on your head.
2. Exhale as you raise your upper body up to around a 45-degree angle, squeezing your abs all the while and keeping your chin off your chest.
3. Inhale as you lower down, trying not to let your abs 'pop' outward. Keep them pulled in.

variation
- Add a twist, add a medicine ball or add pulses.

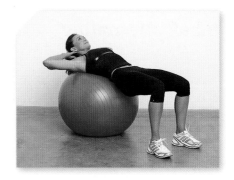

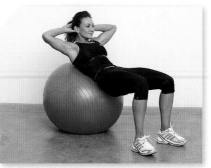

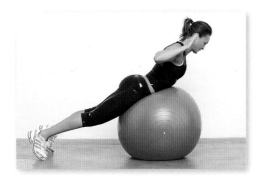

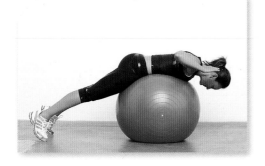

fitball back extension with shoulder blade squeeze

1. Drape yourself over a fitball on your stomach and have your feet either against a wall or your heels tucked under a ledge to support you in position. You can even hold a medicine ball between your feet for support.
2. Place your hands out to the side, similar to a crunch hand position, feeling tension between the shoulder blades.
3. Exhale as you slowly lift your upper body, maintaining a long neck, chin pulled in and squeeze the shoulder blades together at the top.
4. Inhale as you lower and repeat.

variations
- You can hold a medicine ball to your chest as you do this.

fitball alternating back extension

1. Drape yourself over a fitball with your arms straight out in front of you and your legs extended behind.

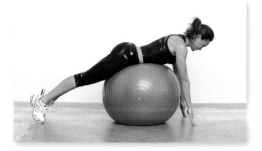

2. Exhale and lift your right arm and your left leg off the floor while your chest should come up and off the ball slightly. You must keep your neck long and your chin pulled in so as not to stress your neck.

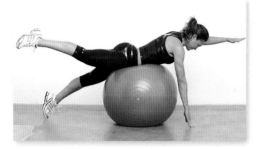

3. Inhale and lower, then repeat on the opposite side.

fitball aeroplane

1. Drape yourself on your stomach over a fitball and have your feet either against a wall or your heels tucked under a ledge to support you in position. You can even hold a medicine ball between your feet for support.
2. Place your arms directly out to the side, feeling tension between the shoulder blades.

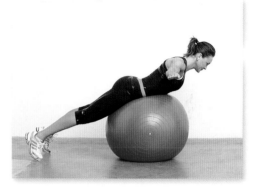

3. Exhale as you slowly lift your upper body, maintaining a long neck, chin pulled in and twisting to one side in 'aeroplane' fashion.

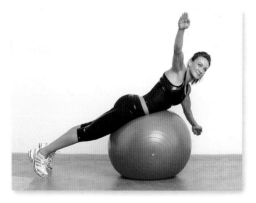

4. Inhale as you twist back to the centre, lower and repeat.

stretching

back stretch

1. Lying on the floor, roll your knees up into your chest and wrap your arms around your legs.
2. Use a towel to wrap around your legs to gently pull them in.

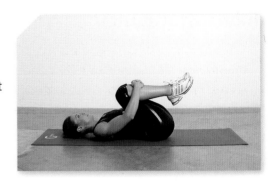

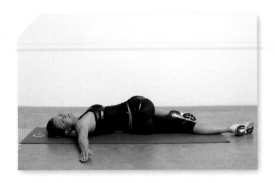

lower back stretch

1. Straighten your legs and lengthen out your body, drawing one knee into the chest. Using the opposite hand, gently pull your knee across your body, gently twisting your lower back.
2. Extend the other arm out, trying to keep both shoulders on the floor. Turn your head away from the knee. Keep breathing and with every exhalation gently sink deeper into the stretch.
3. Repeat on the opposite side.

glute stretch

1. Sit up and cross one leg over the other, keeping the knee pointing out to the side, which will open up your hip. Prop yourself up like you're sitting in a chair by placing your hands behind you and bend the knee of the straight leg.
2. Gradually slide yourself in closer to the crossed leg, maintaining strong upper body posture. Think chest to inside of crossed leg. Be sure to keep your knee out to the side.
3. Repeat on the opposite side.

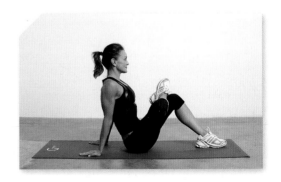

hamstring stretch

1. Extend one leg straight out to the side and bend the other into the centre. Inhale, then exhale as you reach toward your knee, shin, ankle or toes.
2. Keep breathing and working the stretch whilst maintaining strong posture. Aim for a long back and lifted chest.
3. Repeat on the opposite side.

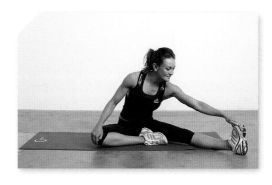

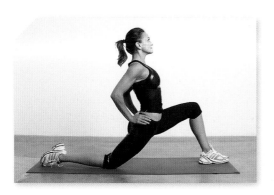

hipflexors

1. Kneeling, step one foot out in front and 'sink' into the position. Aim to lift the chest up and lean slightly back.
2. When you exhale, see if you can sink just that little bit further. If you find this uncomfortable for your knee, roll up a towel and place underneath.
3. Repeat on the opposite side.

inner thigh stretch

These are particularly good if you are doing a lot of running.

1. From all fours, place your hands in front of you for support and extend your leg out to the side with your foot pointing forwards. Your weight should be supported by your bent knee and your hands.
2. Uncurl your back toes and slowly sit your butt back, coming down onto your elbows. Manoeuvre yourself around until you feel the stretch running down the inside of your thigh.
3. Come up on to hands first, then step the leg back in before repeating on the other side.

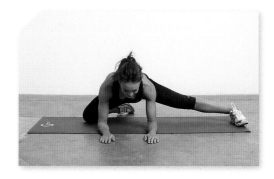

quad stretch

1. Stand up, curl your leg up behind you and grab it with one hand, keeping your knees together. Gently pull your foot into your butt.
2. Stand tall, draw your abs in and pull your shoulders back and down, elevating your chest. Think about tucking your tailbone under to get more of a stretch. If your balance is good, take both hands behind you and hold your foot, fully expand your chest and pull your shoulders back.
3. Repeat on the opposite side.

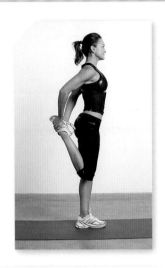

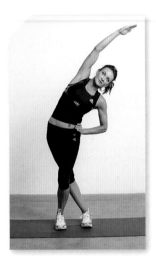

ITB (iliotibial band) stretch

This is a very hard muscle to stretch, and can be tricky for sportsmen and women alike.

1. Stand with your feet hip-width apart, then swing one leg behind the other without twisting your hips. Keep them straight on.
2. Using the same arm as the leg behind, extend and reach, allowing your hips to shift in the opposite direction as you are reaching. Breathe steadily, sinking deeper with every exhalation.
3. Repeat on the opposite side.

chest stretch

1. Still standing, place the palm of your hand onto a wall or pole, and gently turn your self away, opening up one side of your chest.
2. Stand tall, drop your shoulders down and exhale into the stretch.
3. Repeat on the opposite side.

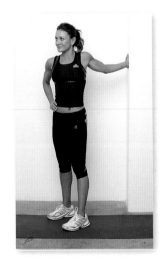

calf stretch

1. Stand facing a solid wall and lean into it like you are trying to push it over.
2. At the same time have one leg back with the toes pointing directly at the wall. This is the key to hitting the calf muscle. Push a little harder on the wall to feel the stretch go deeper.
3. Repeat on the opposite side.

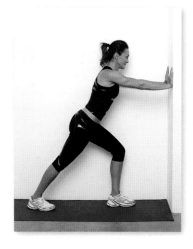

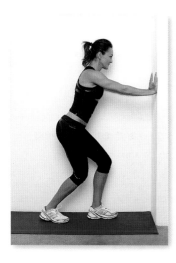

soleus stretch

1. Stand facing a solid wall and lean into it like you are trying to push it over.
2. At the same time, have one leg back with the toes pointing directly at the wall, however, this time the foot is not so far back and you will now bend the knee. The stretch shifts from the belly of the calf muscle to lower down into the soleus. Push a little harder on the wall to feel the stretch go deeper.
3. Repeat on the opposite side.

Acknowledgements

With many thanks to: Maureen Crook, Suellen and David Hughes and Sara Visser for sharing their inspiring weight-loss stories in this book; Nick Wilson and Lisa Cohen for their talented photography; make-up artist Alison Boyle, who also makes a cameo in the fitness test; Kirsten Abbott, Miriam Cannell, Anne Rogan, Arwen Summers and the rest of the Penguin team, especially Adam Laszczuk for the great design; the amazing booksellers for their continued support over the years; Balmain Fitness; and last but not least my wonderful husband Billy who corrects my spelling and keeps me sane.

References

American Chemical Society, 'Revealing Estrogen's Secret Role in Obesity', *Science Daily,* 20 August, 2007, <http://www.sciencedaily.com /releases/2007/08/070820145348.htm>

Andrews, Z., 'Obesity link to killer carbs', *Monash University*, 3 September 2008, <http://www.monash.edu.au/news/monashmemo/stories/20080903/killer-carbs.html>

BBC World News, *Obesity 'Programmed Before Birth'*, 17 November, 2008, <news.bbc.co.uk/2/hi/health/7721438.stm>

Dewey, K., Heinig, M. & Nommsen, L., 'Maternal weight-loss patterns during prolonged lactation', *American Journal of Clinical Nutrition*, vol. 58, no. 2, pp. 162–6, 1993.

Ebrahimi-Mameghani, M., Scott, J.A., Der, G., Lean, M. E. J., & Burns C. M., 'Changes in weight and waist circumference over 9 years in a Scottish population', *European Journal of Clinical Nutrition*, vol. 62, no. 10, pp. 1208–14, doi:10.1038/sj.ejcn.1602839, published online 11 July 2007.

Vesco, K. et. al., 'Excessive Gestational Weight Gain and Postpartum Weight Retention Among Obese Women'; *Obstetrics & Gynecology*, vol. 114, no. 5, pp. 1069–75, November 2009.

Wrotniak, B. H., Shults, J., Butts, S. & Stettler, N., 'Gestational weight gain and risk of overweight in the offspring at age 7', *American Journal of Clinical Nutrition*, vol. 87, no. 6, pp. 1818–24, June 2008.

Index